Idiopathic Generalised Epilepsies

C.P. Panayiotopoulos

Idiopathic Generalised Epilepsies

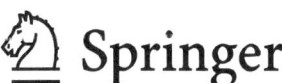 Springer

C.P. Panayiotopoulos M.D., Ph.D., F.R.C.P.
Department of Clinical Neurophysiology and Epilepsies
St Thomas' Hospital
London
United Kingdom

ISBN 978-1-4471-4038-2   ISBN 978-1-4471-4039-9   (eBook)
DOI 10.1007/978-1-4471-4039-9
Springer Dordrecht Heidelberg New York London

Library of Congress Control Number: 2012940656

Printed on acid-free paper

Springer is part of Springer Science+Business Media (www.springer.com)

Preface

The most important milestone in modern epileptology has been the recognition of epileptic syndromes and diseases, most of which are well defined and easy to diagnose. The syndromic diagnosis of epilepsies has significant clinical, prognostic and therapeutic implications. Hence, a syndrome diagnosis of epilepsies is a basic recommendation made by our formal medical bodies in regard to good clinical practice.

Idiopathic generalised epilepsies (IGEs) constitute one-third of all epilepsies. They are genetically determined and affect otherwise normal people of both sexes and all races. IGEs manifest with typical absences, myoclonic jerks and generalised tonic clonic seizures, alone or in varying combinations and severity. Absence status epilepticus is common. Most syndromes of IGE start in childhood or adolescence, but some have an adult onset. They are usually lifelong, though a few such as childhood absence epilepsy are age-related.

The EEG is the most sensitive test in the diagnosis and confirmation of IGE. EEG shows generalised discharges of spikes, polyspikes or spike/polyspike-waves either ictally or interictally. These discharges are often precipitated by hyperventilation, sleep deprivation and intermittent photic stimulation (IPS). Inconspicuous clinical manifestations become apparent on video-EEG and with breath counting during hyperventilation. The EEG is unlikely to be normal in untreated patients. In suspected cases with a normal routine awake EEG, an EEG during sleep and awakening should be obtained.

Molecular genetic analyses have led to important breakthroughs in the identification of candidate genes and loci; genetic heterogeneity is common.

Treatment of IGEs is demanding for two main reasons. First, AEDs beneficial in focal epilepsies are contraindicated in IGEs. Secondly, the efficacy of AEDs differs even within IGE seizures. Most IGEs respond well to appropriate AED, but treatment is often lifelong.

This concise booklet provides a physician-friendly modern review of all syndromes of IGEs, their prevalence, clinical features, EEG manifestations and treatment. Key points of clinical significance are emphasised. The aim is to assist health care professionals in optimising the diagnosis and management of IGEs.

March 2012, Oxford   C.P. Panayiotopoulos, M.D., Ph.D., F.R.C.P.

Contents

Abbreviations

ACTH	Adrenocorticotrophic hormone
ADCME	Autosomal dominant cortical tremor, myoclonus and epilepsy
ADR	Adverse drug reaction
AED	Anti-epileptic drug
CAE	Childhood absence epilepsy
CI	Confidence interval
EEG	Electroencephalogram
EFS+	Epilepsy with febrile seizures plus
EGTCSA	Epilepsy with GTCS on awakening
EM-AS	Epilepsy with myoclonic–astatic seizure
EMEA	European Medicines Agency
EMG	Electromyography
FDA US	Food & Drug Administration
GPSWD	Generalised polyspike–wave discharge
GTCS	Generalised tonic–clonic seizure
HR	Hazard ratio
IGE	Idiopathic generalised epilepsy
ILAE	International League Against Epilepsy
IPS	Intermittent photic stimulation
JAE	Juvenile absence epilepsy
JME	Juvenile myoclonic epilepsy
MCM	Major congenital malformation
MRI	Magnetic resonance imaging
PMA	Perioral myoclonia with absences
RCT	Randomised controlled trial
TAS	Typical absence seizures

Introduction

The idiopathic generalised epilepsies (IGEs) constitute nearly a third of all epilepsies.[1] They are genetically determined and affect otherwise healthy people of both sexes and all races.[2] IGEs manifest with typical absences, myoclonic jerks and generalised tonic–clonic seizures (GTCSs), alone or in varying combinations and severity.[3] Seizure-precipitating factors and photosensitivity are common.[4] Most seizures occur on awakening, particularly after sleep deprivation. Absence status epilepticus is frequent.[5] Syndromes of IGE usually start in childhood or adolescence, but some have an adult onset.[6,7] They are generally life-long, although a few are age-related.

The diagnosis of IGE is usually easy, although IGEs are frequently misdiagnosed as non-epileptic or as other focal and symptomatic epileptic disorders.[8,9] The EEG is the most sensitive test in the diagnosis and confirmation of IGE.[10] The EEG shows generalised polyspike–wave discharges (GPSWD) and/or generalised spike–wave discharges (GSWD), either ictally or inter-ictally. These discharges are frequently precipitated by hyperventilation, sleep deprivation and intermittent photic stimulation (IPS). Inconspicuous clinical manifestations become apparent on video-EEG and with breath counting during hyperventilation. The EEG is unlikely to be normal in untreated patients. In suspected cases with a normal, routine awake EEG, an EEG during sleep and awakening should be obtained. Molecular genetic analyses have led to important breakthroughs in the identification of candidate genes and loci; genetic heterogeneity is common.[2]

Treatment of IGEs with older[11] and newer[12] anti-epileptic drugs (AEDs) is demanding. There are two main reasons for this. First, some AEDs of benefit in focal epilepsies are contraindicated in the IGEs.[13] Second, efficacy of AEDs differs even within seizures of IGEs. IGEs usually respond well to appropriate AEDs, but treatment is often life-long. Advice regarding circadian distribution, lifestyle and seizure precipitants is as important as drug treatment.[14] Avoidance of precipitating factors and adherence to long-term medication is essential to avoid seizures. Children and women with IGEs merit special concern and management. The fact that nearly half of patients with IGEs are currently taking 'ill-advised AED' medication[15,16] is a grave problem that needs to be addressed.[17] Misdiagnosis and inappropriate AED treatment are confounding factors accounting for avoidable intractability, morbidity and sometimes mortality.

The IGEs have been extensively reviewed in an expert multi-authored supplement of Epilepsia,[18] including a thorough historical account by Peter Wolf.[19]

Considerations on Classification

The classification of IGE is controversial. There are two schools of thought with diversely opposing views:

1. IGE is one disease.
2. IGE comprises many distinct syndromes.

In practical terms the view that 'IGE is one disease' would be an overall easy clinical diagnostic approach, but this would discourage diagnostic precision. The view that 'IGE comprises many distinct syndromes' would be more demanding diagnostically, sometimes requiring exhaustive clinical and video-EEG data, but this is often a price that we have to pay as physicians in pursuing accurate diagnosis, which is the golden rule in medicine. This view also (1) satisfies 'maximum practical application to differential diagnosis', which is a main reason for reorganising the classification of epileptic syndromes, and (2) takes advantage of 'significant advances in our understanding' of IGEs, which constitute a third of 'epilepsy'.

Along these lines there is no justification for the proposed unification of 'IGEs with onset in adolescence'.[20] The major conceptual problem in this proposition is that it takes 'age at onset-adolescence' as the most significant, almost defining factor, which is at variance with the definition of a syndrome.[21] Furthermore, the same IGE syndrome may start in childhood, adolescence and occasionally adult life.[21] On the surface, syndromes of IGE may look alike if their clinico-EEG manifestations are not properly analysed. For example, juvenile myoclonic epilepsy (JME) and juvenile absence epilepsy (JAE) both manifest with absences, myoclonic jerks and GTCSs. However, severe absences are the main and the most disturbing seizure type in JAE; myoclonic jerks may not occur or may be randomly distributed. Conversely, myoclonic jerks on awakening are the defining symptom of JME; absences are mild and occur in only a third of patients. In addition, video-EEG studies have documented that the clinico-EEG features of typical absence seizures (TAS) are syndrome-related.[22,23] Unifying all TAS as a single type is of no benefit to any cause.

In genetic terms, animal studies have documented numerous syndromes of IGEs[24] and this is likely to also be the case in humans,[23] where new genetic technologies are rapidly identifying specific genes responsible for IGEs.

Syndromes of IGE Recognised by the ILAE

The following are IGEs as listed in the new ILAE classification scheme[25] in accordance with the age at onset (Table 1.1):

- Benign myoclonic epilepsy in infancy
- Epilepsy with febrile seizures plus (EFS+)
- Epilepsy with myoclonic–astatic seizures (EM-AS)
- Epilepsy with myoclonic absences (MAE)
- Childhood absence epilepsy (CAE)
- IGEs with variable phenotypes
  - Juvenile absence epilepsy (JAE)
  - Juvenile myoclonic epilepsy (JME)
  - Epilepsy with GTCSs only

Video-EEG documentation of many patients with these syndromes can be found in the companion CD of references.[23,26]

Report of 2001[25]	Report of 2006[a,56]
Idiopathic focal epilepsies in infancy and childhood	*Neonatal period*
Benign infantile seizures (non-familial)	Benign familial neonatal seizures (3) – probably a disease
Benign childhood epilepsy with centrotemporal spikes	Early myoclonic encephalopathy (3)
Early onset benign childhood occipital epilepsy (Panayiotopoulos type)	Ohtahara syndrome (3)
Late-onset childhood occipital epilepsy (Gastaut type)	*Infancy*
Familial (autosomal dominant) focal epilepsies	Migrating partial seizures of infancy (3) – now recognised as a syndrome
Autosomal dominant nocturnal frontal lobe epilepsy	West syndrome (3)
Benign familial neonatal seizures	Myoclonic epilepsy in infancy (3) – the word benign has been removed
Benign familial infantile seizures	Benign infantile seizures (3) – now familial and non-familial forms are combined

Table 1.1 Epileptic syndromes in the ILAE Task Force report

Report of 2001[25]	Report of 2006[a,56]
Familial temporal lobe epilepsy	Dravet syndrome (3)
Familial focal epilepsy with variable foci[b]	Myoclonic encephalopathy in non-progressive disorders (3) – now recognised as a syndrome
Symptomatic and probably symptomatic epilepsies	*Childhood*
Limbic epilepsies:	Early onset benign childhood occipital epilepsy (Panayiotopoulos type) (3)
Mesial temporal lobe epilepsy with hippocampal sclerosis	Epilepsy with myoclonic–astatic seizures (3)
Mesial temporal lobe epilepsy defined by specific aetiologies	Benign childhood epilepsy with centrotemporal spikes (3)
Other types defined by location and aetiology	Late-onset childhood occipital epilepsy (Gastaut type) (1)
Neocortical epilepsies:	Epilepsy with myoclonic absences (2)
Rasmussen syndrome	Lennox–Gastaut syndrome (3)
Hemiconvulsion–hemiplegia syndrome	Epileptic encephalopathy with continuous spikes and waves during sleep, including Landau–Kleffner syndrome (3) – the two are now combined
Other types defined by location and aetiology	Childhood absence epilepsy (3)
Migrating partial seizures of early infancy[b]	*Adolescence*
Idiopathic generalised epilepsies	Juvenile absence epilepsy (3)
Benign myoclonic epilepsy in infancy	Juvenile myoclonic epilepsy (3)
Epilepsy with myoclonic–astatic seizures	Progressive myoclonus epilepsies (3) – diseases rather than syndromes
Childhood absence epilepsy	*Less specific age relationship*
Epilepsy with myoclonic absences	Autosomal dominant nocturnal frontal lobe epilepsy (3)
Idiopathic generalised epilepsies with variable phenotypes:	Familial temporal lobe epilepsies (3)
Juvenile absence epilepsy	Mesial temporal lobe epilepsy with hippocampal sclerosis (2) – probably more than one syndrome
Juvenile myoclonic epilepsy	Rasmussen syndrome (3) – disease or syndrome?
Epilepsy with GTCSs only	Gelastic seizures with hypothalamic hamartoma (3) – probably a disease
Generalised epilepsies with febrile seizures plus[b]	*Special epilepsy conditions*
Reflex epilepsies	Symptomatic focal epilepsies not otherwise specified
Idiopathic photosensitive occipital lobe epilepsy	Epilepsy with GTCSs only – unable to agree on any syndrome with this feature; whether EGTCSW exists is unclear
Other visual sensitive epilepsies	Reflex epilepsies (unclear if other reflex epilepsies constitute syndromes):

Table 1.1 (continued)

Report of 2001[25]	Report of 2006[a,56]
Primary reading epilepsy	Idiopathic photosensitive occipital lobe epilepsy (2)
Startle epilepsy	Primary reading epilepsy (3)
Epileptic encephalopathies	Hot water epilepsy in infants (2)
Early myoclonic encephalopathy	Febrile seizures plus (FS+) (part of generalised epilepsy with FS+, which is broader than a single generalised syndrome)
Ohtahara syndrome	Familial focal epilepsy with variable foci (3) – now recognised as a syndrome
West syndrome	*Conditions with epileptic seizures that do not require a diagnosis of epilepsy*
Dravet syndrome (previously known as severe myoclonic epilepsy in infancy)	Benign neonatal seizures (2)
Myoclonic status in non-progressive encephalopathies*	Febrile seizures (3)
Lennox–Gastaut syndrome	*Categories that might be considered in future classification systems*
Landau–Kleffner syndrome	Autosomal dominant epilepsies
Epilepsy with continuous spike–waves during slow-wave sleep	Epileptic encephalopathies
Progressive myoclonus epilepsies	Generalised epilepsy with FS+
See specific diseases	Idiopathic generalised epilepsies
Seizures not necessarily requiring a diagnosis of epilepsy	Idiopathic focal epilepsies
Benign neonatal seizures	Reflex epilepsies
Febrile seizures	
Reflex seizures	
Alcohol-withdrawal seizures	
Drug or other chemically induced seizures	
Immediate and early post-traumatic seizures	
Single seizures or isolated clusters of seizures	
Rarely repeated seizures (oligoepilepsy)	

Table adapted with permission from Engel (2001)[25] and Engel (2006)[56]

[a]The epilepsy syndromes listed were individually discussed by the Core Group and rated on a score of 1–3 (3 being the most clearly and reproducibly defined) regarding the certainty with which the group believed each syndrome represented a unique diagnostic entity. EGTCSW, epilepsy with GTCSs on awakening.
[b]Syndromes in development

Table 1.1 (continued)

Epilepsy with Myoclonic–Astatic Seizures

Synonym: EM-AS, Doose syndrome.

EM-AS[23,27-36] is considered as an IGE in the new ILAE diagnostic scheme.[25] The diagnosis of this syndrome requires careful application of inclusion and exclusion criteria (Table 2.1). Its characteristic symptom, myoclonic–astatic seizures, is shared by many other childhood syndromes, particularly epileptic encephalopathies.

Considerations on Classification

The new ILAE Task Force considers EM-AS as an IGE,[25] a view which is similar to that of Doose[29]:

> *EM-AS belongs to the epilepsies with primarily generalised seizures and thus stands in one line with absence epilepsies, JME, as well as the infantile and juvenile idiopathic epilepsy with GTCS. Like these types of epilepsy, EM-AS is polygenically determined with little non-genetic variability. The disease is characterised by the following criteria: genetic predisposition (high incidence of seizures and/or genetic EEG patterns in relatives); mostly normal development and no neurological deficits before onset; primarily generalised myoclonic, astatic or myoclonic–astatic seizures, short absences and mostly GTCSs; no tonic seizures or tonic drop attacks during daytime (except for some rare cases with a most unfavourable course); generalised EEG patterns (spikes and waves, photosensitivity, 4–7 Hz rhythms), no multifocal EEG-abnormalities (but often pseudofoci).*
>
> *–Doose[29] on EM-AS*

Inclusion criteria
Normal development prior to the onset of seizures and normal MRI
Onset of myoclonic, myoclonic–atonic or atonic seizures between 7 months and 6 years of age
Normal background EEG with 2–3 Hz GPSWD without focal spike discharges
Exclusion criteria
Dravet syndrome, Lennox–Gastaut syndrome, myoclonic epilepsy in infancy or other epileptic syndromes manifesting with myoclonic–atonic seizures
Tonic seizures

Table 2.1 Diagnostic criteria for idiopathic EM-AS[29,30]

C.P. Panayiotopoulos, *Idiopathic Generalised Epilepsies*,
DOI 10.1007/978-1-4471-4039-9_2, © Springer-Verlag London 2012

This contrasts markedly with the previous classification of 1989 where EM-AS was listed as a 'cryptogenic/symptomatic' generalised epilepsy in the same group of disorders as that of the Lennox–Gastaut syndrome.[21]

The problem may reflect a lack of specific criteria and undefined boundaries of certain epileptic syndromes and particularly the epileptic encephalopathies, which may manifest with myoclonic–astatic seizures. This particularly refers to Dravet syndrome, Lennox–Gastaut syndrome and atypical benign partial epilepsy of childhood. Cases of benign and severe myoclonic epilepsy in infants may have been included in EM-AS.[29] Other myoclonic epilepsies with brief seizures reported as intermediate cases between EM-AS and Lennox–Gastaut syndrome probably prove this point.[37]

However, it is generally accepted that some children with myoclonic–astatic seizures are otherwise normal with no discernible causes other than a strong genetic epileptic background and these probably represent the genuine, idiopathic syndrome of EM-AS (of Doose syndrome to distinguish them from symptomatic or cryptogenic epilepsies with myoclonic–astatic seizures). Kaminska et al.[38] found evidence that EM-AS is distinct from Lennox–Gastaut syndrome, 'and the distinction appears from the first year of the disorder'.

Another important point to remember is that this syndrome mainly manifests with myoclonic–atonic seizures and these are not synonymous with myoclonic–astatic seizures.

Demographic Data

Prevalence may be about 1–2 % of all childhood epilepsies; two-thirds are boys. Onset is between 7 months and 6 years (peak 2–4 years).

Clinical Manifestations

EM-AS is characterised by myoclonic–astatic seizures that often occur together with atonic, myoclonic and absence seizures; myoclonic–astatic status epilepticus is common.

Children are normal prior to the onset of seizures. In two-thirds, febrile and afebrile GTCSs appear first, several months prior to the onset of myoclonic–astatic seizures.

Myoclonic–astatic (in fact, myoclonic–atonic) seizures are the defining symptoms (100 % of the cases).[29] These manifest with symmetrical myoclonic jerks immediately followed by loss of muscle tone (post-myoclonic atonia; Fig. 2.1).

In addition, atonic and absence seizures occur frequently, sometimes many times per day in the active period of the disease.

Atonic seizures of sudden, brief and severe loss of postural tone may involve the whole body or only the head. Attacks are brief, 1–4 s and frequent. Generalised loss of postural tone causes a lightning-like fall. The patient collapses on the floor irresistibly. In brief and milder attacks there is only head nodding or bending of the knees.

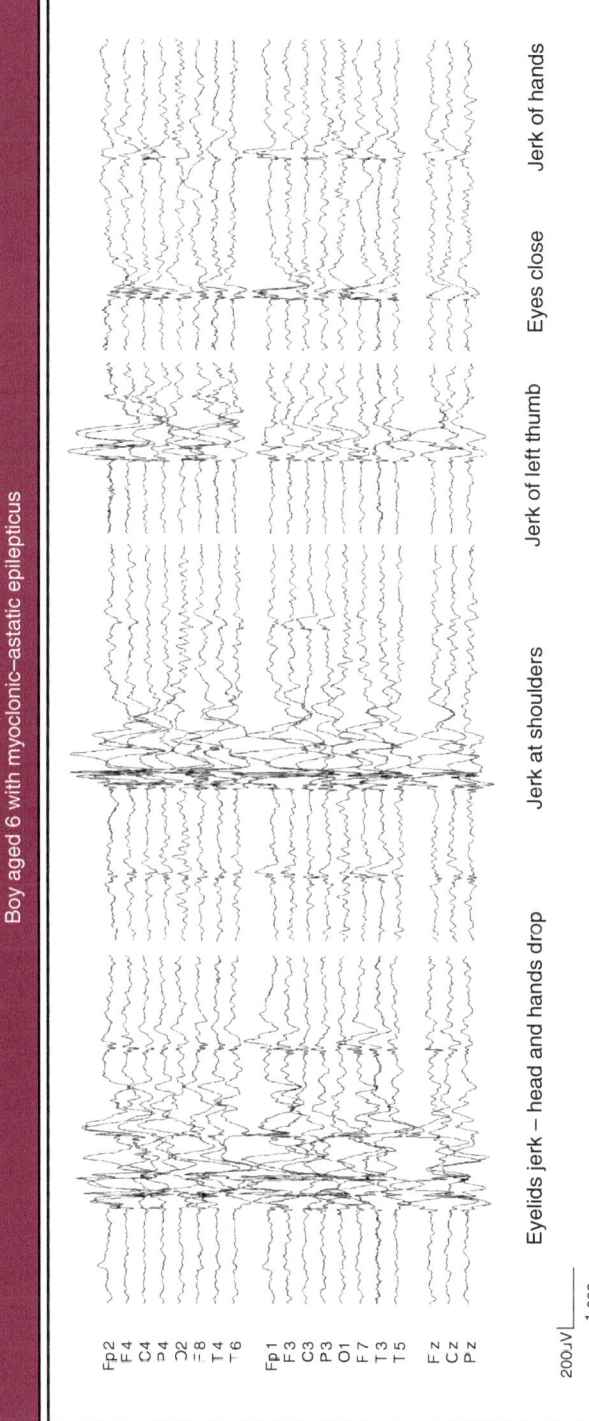

Boy aged 6 with myoclonic–astatic epilepticus

Eyelids jerk – head and hands drop   Jerk at shoulders   Jerk of left thumb   Eyes close   Jerk of hands

200 μV

1 sec

Fig. 2.1 Samples from video-EEG of a 6-year-old normal boy with EM-AS. The background activity was normal but there were frequent (at least every 10 s) 3–6 Hz GPSWD with anterior maximum They were brief for 1–4 s. These were frequently associated with single jerks of mainly the shoulders but also, on other occasions, of the thumb or eyelids. The jerks occurred simultaneously with the first or the second polyspike–wave complex of the discharges. Some jerks were followed by atonic attacks. The EEG also showed brief (<0.5 s) abortive 1.5 Hz GPSWD with anterior maximum and an alternating but not consistent side emphasis. There were no clinical manifestations. The paroxysmal discharges occurred with eyes opened and closed, spontaneously and during overbreathing. IPS did not evoke photoparoxysmal responses

Myoclonic jerks precede or less often intersperse with the atonic manifestations (Fig. 2.1).

Absence seizures alone without clinical symptoms, other than impairment of consciousness, are exceptional. However, more than half of the cases have brief absence seizures often together with myoclonic jerks, facial myoclonias and atonic manifestations.

Tonic seizures are an exclusion criterion.

Non-convulsive status epilepticus (myoclonic–atonic status epilepticus) lasting for hours or even days (Fig. 2.2) is common, affecting a third of patients. This manifests with varying degrees of usually severe cognitive impairment or cloudiness of consciousness interspersed with repetitive myoclonic and atonic fits. Facial myoclonus of eyelids and mouth may be continuous, together with irregular jerks of the limbs and atonic seizures of head nodding or falls. Myoclonic–atonic status epilepticus may occur several times during a period of 1 or 2 years.

Aetiology

EM-AS may be genetically determined in a multifactorial polygenic fashion with variable penetrance.[27,29,34] A third of patients have familial seizure disorders and mainly IGEs.[27,29,34] Of significant interest are the clinical and molecular studies of EFS+, where myoclonic–atonic seizures are common.[31] EFS+ has strong genetic links with Dravet syndrome. However, mutations in the SCN1A gene are rarely found in patients with EM–AS.[31,38] Five percent of patients with EM-AS have SLC2A1 mutations with GLUT-1 deficiency and require treatment with ketogenic diet.[39]

Diagnostic Procedures

By definition all tests other than EEG are normal.

Electroencephalography

Inter-ictal EEG may be normal at the stage of febrile or afebrile GTCSs. Rhythmic theta activity in the parasagittal regions may be the only significant abnormality. Subsequently, when myoclonic–atonic seizures appear, there are frequent clusters of 2 or 3 Hz GPSWD interrupted by high-amplitude slow waves in cases with predominant atonic or myoclonic–atonic seizures. In children with predominantly myoclonic seizures, paroxysms of irregular spikes or polyspike–wave complexes prevail.

The *ictal EEG* of myoclonic and atonic seizures manifests with discharges of irregular spike–wave or polyspike–wave complexes at a frequency of 2.5–3 Hz or more (Figs. 2.1 and 2.2). Atonia is usually concurrent with the slow wave of a single or polyspike–wave complex, and the intensity of the atonia is proportional to the amplitude of the slow wave. Drop attacks are

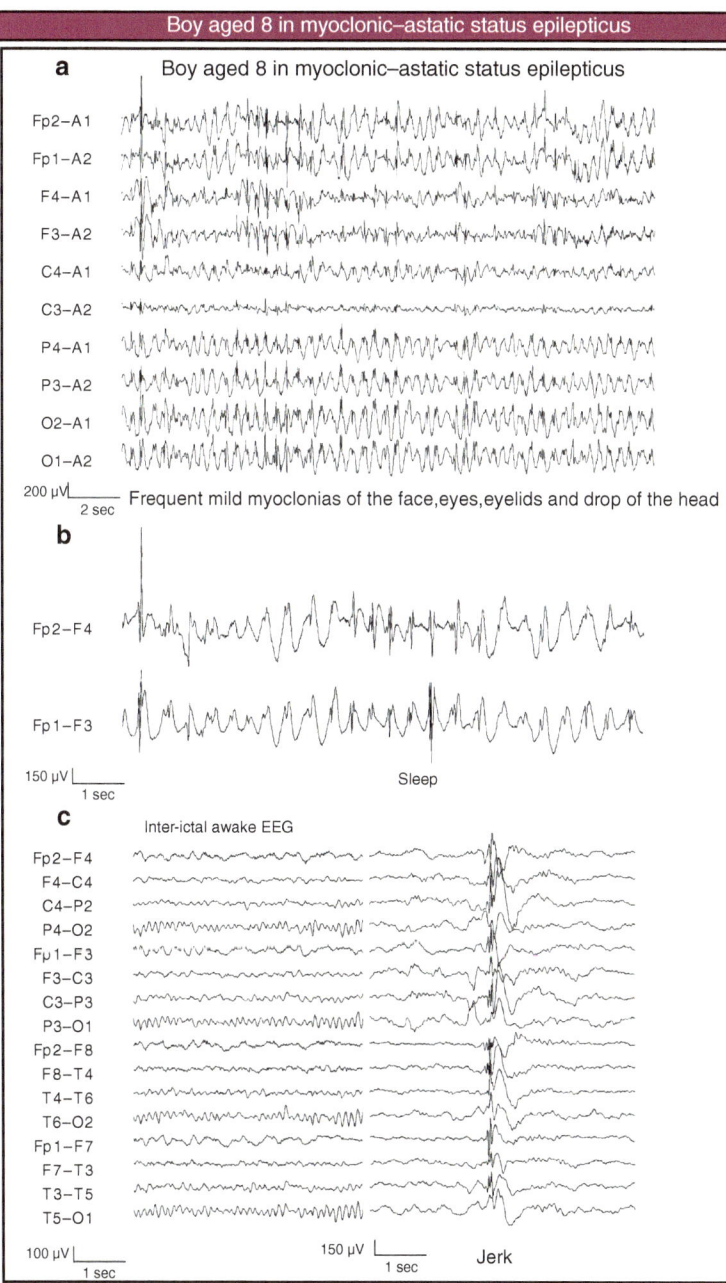

Fig. 2.2 Samples of video-EEG of a boy in myoclonic–astatic status epilepticus. (**a**) The EEG showed electrical status epilepticus during wakefulness and sleep. This consisted of nearly continuous 2.5–3 Hz GPSWD. This pattern occasionally alternated with relatively normal background activity lasting <30 s. The main clinical manifestations were frequent facial subtle myoclonias (eyelid fluttering, upwards deviation of the eyes with spontaneous eye opening associated with fast eyelid fluttering, subtle facial twitches) and a few massive myoclonic jerks occasionally with some atonic components. Clinically, there was no apparent impairment of consciousness. (**b**) Details of the EEG shown in (**a**) (note calibration: higher sensitivity and faster speed). (**c**) The video-EEG 1 month later was normal during wakefulness with a few myoclonic jerks only during sleep

associated with diffuse electromyography (EMG) paucity indicating their true atonic nature.[30] The myoclonus of EM-AS appears to be a primarily generalised epileptic phenomenon, which differs from that of Lennox–Gastaut syndrome,[40] which originates from the frontal cortex spreading to contralateral and ipsilateral cortical areas.

In myoclonic–atonic status epilepticus, the EEG shows continuous or discontinuous and repetitive 2–3 Hz GPSWD (Fig. 2.2).

Differential Diagnosis

Differential diagnosis of EM-AS is mainly between benign myoclonic epilepsy in infancy, Dravet syndrome, Lennox–Gastaut syndrome and late-onset West syndrome. In general, children with EM-AS are normal prior to the develop-

Diagnostic Tips

The diagnosis of EM-AS is probably secured if myoclonic–atonic seizures start in a previously normal child with pre-existing febrile or afebrile GTCSs and familial seizure disorders (see, however, EFS+).[31]

Differential diagnostic problems from Lennox–Gastaut syndrome probably reflect ill-defined inclusion and exclusion criteria.

ment of seizures, have a strong family history of IGE, and the background EEG and brain imaging are normal.

Progressive myoclonic epilepsies, such as myoclonic epilepsy with ragged red fibres, Lafora and Unverricht disease, may initially imitate EM-AS. However, their associated relevant neurological abnormalities and, often, their relentless progression and deterioration will establish the diagnosis.

Atypical benign partial epilepsy of childhood may also imitate EM-AS, because of repeated falls, absences and diffuse slow-spike–wave activity mainly in the sleep EEG. The main differentiating point is that these children also have nocturnal focal seizures similar to the rolandic seizures that are often the presenting symptom. Also, the EEG shows centrotemporal and other functional spikes in various locations.

Atypical evolutions of rolandic epilepsy[41,42] *and Panayiotopoulos syndrome*[43,44] may present with similar features as EM-AS, but these follow the typical presentations of these syndromes. A similar, but reversible, clinico-EEG condition may be induced by carbamazepine,[45] oxcarbazepine[46] and lamotrigine[47] in a few children with rolandic seizures or Panayiotopoulos syndrome.[48] This possibility should be considered in children with benign focal seizures and dramatic deterioration after treatment with these AEDs.

Children with 'epilepsy with continuous spike-and-wave during sleep' may also have drop attacks due to atypical absences or negative myoclonus.

Non-epileptic myoclonus may rarely raise a diagnostic problem with EM-AS.

Prognosis

Prognosis is unclear, probably because of different inclusion and exclusion criteria. Half of patients achieve a seizure-free state and normal or near-normal development. These may correspond to the idiopathic form of EM-AS (of Doose syndrome). Spontaneous remission with normal development has been observed in a few untreated cases but these may belong to myoclonic epilepsy in infancy. The others, probably belonging to symptomatic or cryptogenic cases or other syndromes, continue with seizures, severe impairment of cognitive functions and behavioural abnormalities. Ataxia, poor motor function, dysarthria and poor language development may emerge.

Management

Drug therapy is dictated by the type of seizure. Valproate, which is effective in myoclonic jerks, atonic seizures and absences, is the most efficacious of the AEDs. Add-on small doses of lamotrigine have a beneficial pharmacodynamic interaction with valproate. Topiramate reduces the frequency of atonic seizures[49] and levetiracetam may be an effective therapeutic option.[12,50]

In resistant cases, ketogenic diet, alone[51] or followed by adrenocorticotrophic hormone (ACTH) and ethosuximide, have been found to be highly beneficial.[52] Benzodiazepines, acetazolamide, sulthiame and even bromides are also used.

Carbamazepine, phenytoin and vigabatrin are contraindicated (Table 13.2).

In myoclonic–atonic status epilepticus, intravenous benzodiazepines are often efficacious, but may, rarely, precipitate tonic status epilepticus.

Childhood Absence Epilepsy

CAE[23,53,54] is the prototype IGE of typical absence seizures (TAS).[55] It is genetically determined, age related and affects otherwise normal children. Table 3.1 lists inclusion and exclusion criteria.

Considerations on Classification

The ILAE Commission of 1989[21] defines CAE by age at onset and the frequency of absences:

> *CAE (pyknolepsy) occurs in children of school age (peak manifestation age 6–7 years), with a strong genetic predisposition in otherwise normal children. It appears more frequently in girls than in boys. It is characterised by very frequent (several to many per day) absences. The EEG reveals bilateral, synchronous symmetrical spike–waves, usually 3 Hz, on a normal background activity. During adolescence, GTCSs often develop. Otherwise, absences may remit or more rarely, persist as the only seizure type.*[21]

Inclusion criteria for CAE
Age at onset between 4 and 10 years and a peak at 5–7 years
Normal neurological state and development
Brief (4–20 s, exceptionally longer) and frequent (tens per day) absence seizures with abrupt and severe impairment (loss) of consciousness. Automatisms are frequent but have no significance in the diagnosis
EEG ictal generalised discharges of high-amplitude spike and double or maximum triple spike and slow-wave complexes. They are rhythmic at around 3 Hz with a gradual and regular slowdown from the initial to the terminal phase of the discharge. Their duration varies from 4 to 20 s (exceptionally longer)
Exclusion criteria for CAE
The following may be incompatible with CAE:
Other types of seizure, such as GTCSs, or myoclonic jerks prior to or during the active stage of absences
Eyelid myoclonia, perioral myoclonia, rhythmic massive limb jerking, and single or arrhythmic myoclonic jerks of the head, trunk or limbs. However, mild myoclonic elements of the eyes, eyebrows and eyelids may be featured – particularly in the first 3 s of the absence seizure
Mild or no impairment of consciousness during the 3 Hz discharges
Brief EEG 3 Hz spike–wave paroxysms of <4 s, polyspikes (more than three) or ictal discharge fragmentations
Visual (photic) and other sensory precipitation of clinical seizures

Reproduced from Loiseau and Panayiotopoulos[54]

Table 3.1 Inclusion and exclusion criteria for CAE

C.P. Panayiotopoulos, *Idiopathic Generalised Epilepsies*,
DOI 10.1007/978-1-4471-4039-9_3, © Springer-Verlag London 2012

The new ILAE reports initially classified CAE as an IGE,[25] but later simply listed it among other syndromes of childhood (Table 1.1).[56]

The ILAE definition[21] is very broad and requires revision.[55] Otherwise, any type of frequent absence seizures occurring in childhood would be erroneously equated with CAE. Because of this ambiguity, the epidemiology, genetics, age at onset, clinical manifestations, other types of seizure, long-term prognosis and the treatment of CAE that are reviewed in this chapter may not accurately reflect the syndrome of CAE. It is also because of this ambiguity that some authors: (1) have divided patients with childhood-onset absence seizures into 'sub-syndromes', including those who remit, those who persist into adolescence and develop GTCSs, and those who develop both GTCSs and myoclonic seizures during adolescence[57]; and (2) consider that CAE 'evolves' into JAE or JME.[58]

The inclusion and exclusion criteria of Table 3.1 proposed by Loiseau and Panayiotopoulos[54] for CAE should not be taken as an extreme position. They do not differ significantly from the ILAE[21] criteria of CAE with:

- Age at onset in childhood
- Very frequent (several to many per day) absences, presumably with severe impairment of consciousness
- Ictal EEG with bilateral, synchronous and symmetrical 3 Hz GSWD, on a normal background activity (that presumably excludes fragmented, asymmetrical and asynchronous 3–5 Hz GSWD with intra-discharge variations)
- GTCSs accepted only if they develop later in adolescence.

Also, the ILAE Commission,[21] by accepting 'epilepsy with myoclonic absences' as a separate syndrome, differentiates myoclonic absences from typical absences of CAE. It is along this line that eyelid myoclonia (which is a predominantly myoclonic and less of an absence syndrome) is counted as an exclusion criterion. Whether perioral myoclonia or single violent jerks during the ictus of an absence seizure is an exclusion criterion may be debatable. However, their presence indicates a worse prognosis (see relevant syndromes). The same applies to polyspikes (more than three spikes per wave), which also indicate a bad prognosis,[57,59] or the coexistence of myoclonic jerks or GTCSs.[22]

Furthermore, by accepting 'typical absence seizures consistently provoked by specific stimuli' as a specific type of reflex seizures, the ILAE Commission[21] indicates that these may be a separate group from CAE.

A recent report on CAE[60] well reflects the misunderstanding surrounding this syndrome (Table 3.2). It is used here as an example to emphasise the points made in this chapter and for the differentiation of IGEs with absence seizures in general[55]:

- The report defines TAS 'as a clinical change associated with generalised spike-and-slow-wave activity or multiple-spike-and-slow-wave activity with a frequency of >2.5 Hz at onset'. Whether this clinical change always involved impairment of consciousness is not stated. Impairment

Electroclinical features[a]	No. of patients	Epileptic syndromes that these features are more likely to manifest	Exclusion criterion of CAE?
A. Duration of seizure <4s	21	JME, EMA1	Yes
B. Age of child <4 years	7	EMA, PMA, MAE	Probably yes (exceptional)
C. No severe impairment of consciousness during	16	All other IGEs with seizure absences but CAE and JAE	Yes
D. Myoclonic features in seizures consistent except mild in eyes eyebrows and eyelids	12	MAE, MAE, EMA	Yes if severe and, during the absence†
E. Photic induction of seizures	8	EMA, IGE with photosensitivity	Yes if this is a consistent provocation of clinical seizures
F. More than three spikes	13	JME, EMA	Probably yes if consistent in the per wave whole duration of the discharge†
G. Disorganised discharges	25	JME, PMA, EMA	Yes if consistent in the whole duration of the discharge[b]

[a]The electroclinical features listed were used by Sadleir et al.[60] to define CAE

[b]Onset of absences (first 1 or 2 s) used by the authors for the measurement of the frequency of spike–wave discharges is usually unreliable to make this and other assessments because of variable clinical and EEG manifestations that do not persist in the remainder of the ictal discharge (Fig. 3.1).[22] The same patient may have different onsets of consecutive absences even within the same EEG. Myoclonic jerks, disorganised discharges, more than three spikes per spike–wave complex and fast or slow spike–wave can all occur in the first second of absence seizures in CAE. In accordance with well-documented video-EEG studies, JME is likely to have features A, C, F and G; epilepsy with myoclonic absences (MAE) or perioral myoclonia with absences (PMA) certainly have D; and eyelid myoclonia with absences (EMA) has A–G

Table 3.2 Electroclinical features of a heterogeneous group of children thought to have CAE[60]

of consciousness (absence) is a prerequisite of any definition of TAS. This may be associated with other clinical symptoms (myoclonic, atonic, clonic, autonomic), but these do not constitute TAS without clinically detectable impairment of consciousness.

- The diagnostic criteria for CAE applied in the report are clearly different, not only from those in Table 3.1, but also from the 1989 ILAE definition[21]; the age range was lowered to include children as young as 2 or 3 years old and the seizure frequency was broadened to include 'daily' absences, but not 'several per day' (i.e. pyknolepsy).
- No follow-up is provided despite the original presentation of the patients between 1992 and 1997. It is to be expected that most of them will now be in remission (as for 'true' CAE) or will have developed the full features of other IGEs and conditions with absences starting in childhood, as suggested in Table 3.2.[55]

Demographic Data

Onset is between 4 and 10 years of age (peak at 5–7 years). Two-thirds are girls. Prevalence is about 10% and annual incidence rate is approximately 7/100,000 of children with epileptic seizures younger than 15 or 16 years of age.

Clinical Manifestations

CAE manifests with the most classical example of TAS.[55,61] Absences are severe and frequent, with tens or hundreds per day (hence the term pyknolepsy).[62] They are of abrupt onset and abrupt termination (Fig. 3.1). Their duration varies from 4 to 20 s, although most of them last around 10 s. Clinically, the hallmark of the absence is abrupt, brief and severe impairment of consciousness with unresponsiveness and interruption of the ongoing voluntary activity, which is not restored during the ictus. The eyes spontaneously open, overbreathing, speech and other voluntary activity stops within the first 3 s from the onset of the ictal electrical discharge. Automatisms occur in two-thirds of the seizures but are not stereotyped. The eyes stare or move slowly. Mild myoclonic elements of the eyes, eyebrows and eyelids may feature in CAE in the first 1–3 s of the absence. However, more severe and sustained myoclonic jerks of facial muscles may indicate other IGEs with absences.

The attack ends as abruptly as it has commenced, with sudden resumption of the pre-absence activity as if it had not been interrupted. TAS are nearly invariably provoked by hyperventilation.

Other seizures are not compatible with CAE. The only exception is febrile convulsions prior to the onset of absences and solitary or infrequent GTCSs long after the onset of TAS (usually in adolescence after absences have remitted).

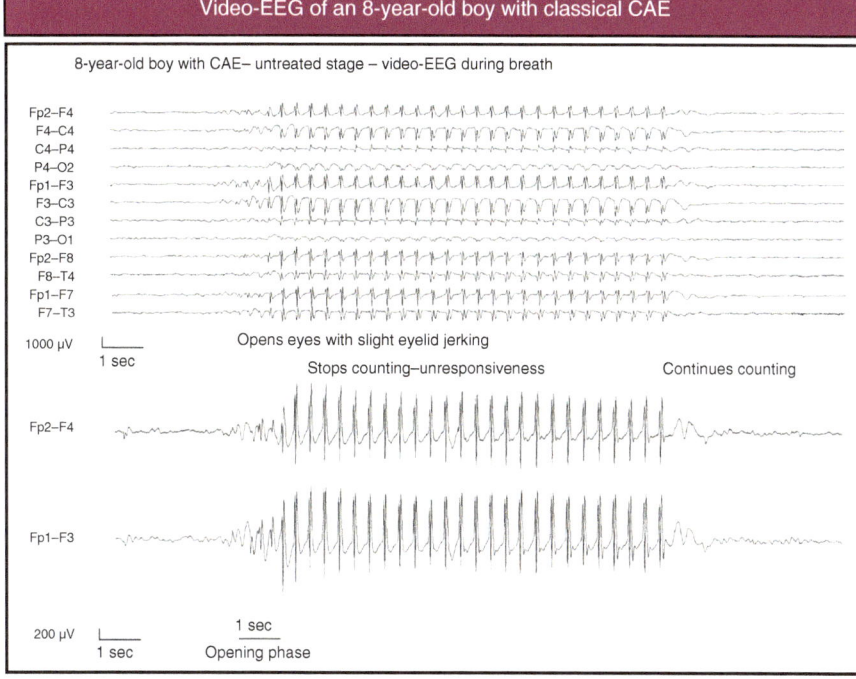

Video-EEG of an 8-year-old boy with classical CAE

8-year-old boy with CAE– untreated stage – video-EEG during breath

Fp2–F4
F4–C4
C4–P4
P4–O2
Fp1–F3
F3–C3
C3–P3
P3–O1
Fp2–F8
F8–T4
Fp1–F7
F7–T3

1000 µV
1 sec

Opens eyes with slight eyelid jerking

Stops counting–unresponsiveness   Continues counting

Fp2–F4

Fp1–F3

200 µV
1 sec

1 sec
1 sec   Opening phase

Fig. 3.1 He was referred for an EEG because of 'blanks and day dreaming'. The diagnosis had been overlooked despite frequent absences for 2 years, which also interfered with his scholastic performance. The illustrated seizure had all the characteristic features of typical absences in CAE. Initially there was some brief eyelid flickering in the opening phase of the GSWD followed by opening of the eyes, eyes and head deviating upwards and to the right, and simultaneous cessation of breath counting. He remained unresponsive during the rest of the GSWD. Counting was restored immediately after the end of the GSWD. Note the fast and asymmetrical onset of the GSWD in the opening phase during the first second. Subsequently, the GSWD was entirely rhythmical and regular with abrupt termination to clinical and EEG normality

Aetiology

Although CAE is genetically determined, the precise mode of inheritance and the genes involved remain largely unidentified.[2,63] In monozygotic twins, 84% had 3 Hz GSWD and only 75% of pairs had clinical absence seizures. These events occurred 16 times more often than in dizygotic twins.[64]

Recently, loci at various chromosomes (1p, 8q24, 5q31.1 and 19p13.2) have been identified in families with absences of childhood onset (not necessarily equated with CAE). Furthermore, current evidence suggests that mutations in genes encoding GABA receptors[65] or brain-expressed voltage-dependent calcium channels[66,67] may underlie CAE.

Acquired factors may play a facilitating role.

Diagnostic Procedures

In typical cases, only EEG is needed.

Electroencephalography

Inter-ictal EEG in CAE has normal background, with frequent rhythmic posterior delta activity, which may be a good prognostic sign.[68] Focal spikes are common.[45,69]

Diagnostic Tips

TAS of CAE are easy to diagnose and reproduce by hyperventilation
Any child with sudden, brief and transient cessation of physical and mental activity should be tested clinically for absences with the hyperventilation test and the events should be video-recorded.

Clinical Tip

In practical terms, a child suspected of typical absences should be asked to overbreathe for 3 min, counting his or her breaths while standing with hands extended in front. Hyperventilation will provoke an absence in more than 90% of those with typical absences. This procedure should preferably be videotaped to document the clinical manifestations. It may reveal features favouring a specific epileptic syndrome and, therefore, may determine the long-term prognosis and management. Video-EEG documentation may be particularly useful if absences prove resistant to treatment, if other seizures develop or for future genetic counselling. Focal spike abnormalities and asymmetrical onset of the ictal GSWD are common and may be a cause of misdiagnosis, particularly in resistant cases. If video-EEG is not available, documentation of absences using a camcorder, mobile phone or modern digital means of recording is recommended.

Ictal discharges consist of 3 Hz GSWD. Spikes are single, double or occasionally triple in the spike and slow-wave complexes (Fig. 3.1).[22] The GSWD are rhythmic at around 3 Hz (2.5–4 Hz), with a gradual and regular slow down of the frequency by 0.5–1 Hz from the initial to the terminal phase of the discharge. The opening phase of the discharge, 1 or 2 s from the onset, is usually fast and unreliable for these measurements. There are no marked variations in the relation of spike to slow wave, no fluctuations in the intradischarge frequency and certainly no fragmentations of the ictal discharges (Fig. 3.1).

Differential Diagnosis

CAE should be the easiest type of epileptic syndrome to diagnose because seizures have abrupt onset and termination, have daily frequency and are nearly invariably provoked by hyperventilation. A child suspected of typical

	Typical absences	**Complex focal seizures**
Clinical criteria		
Duration < 30 s	As a rule	Exceptional
Duration > 1 min	Exceptional	As a rule
Non-convulsive status epilepticus	Frequent	Rare
Daily frequency	As a rule	Rare
Simple automatisms	Frequent	Frequent
Complex behavioural automatisms	Exceptional	Frequent
Simple and complex hallucinations or illusions	Exceptional	Frequent
Bilateral facial myoclonic jerks or eyelid closures	Frequent	Exceptional
Evolving to other focal seizure manifestations	Never	Frequent
Sudden onset and termination	As a rule	Frequent
Post-ictal symptoms	Never	Frequent
Reproduced by hyperventilation	As a rule	Exceptional
Elicited by photic stimulation	Frequent	Exceptional
EEG criteria		
Ictal generalised 3–4 Hz spike and wave	Exclusive	Never
Inter-ictal generalised discharges	Frequent	Exceptional
Inter-ictal focal abnormalities of slow waves	Rare	Frequent
Normal EEG in untreated state	Exceptional	Frequent

The primary differences are shown in red

Table 3.3 Differential diagnosis of typical absences from complex focal seizures

absences should be asked to perform the hyperventilation test as this will provoke an absence in as many as 90% of those who suffer from it.

> *CAE is not synonymous with any type of absence seizures starting in childhood. Therefore, other epilepsy syndromes with absence seizures that may be life-long and have a worse prognosis should be meticulously differentiated from CAE.*

Diagnosis should improve with heightened awareness and video-EEG studies. Exclusion criteria for CAE are significant (Tables 3.1 and 3.2).

Automatisms have no significance in the diagnosis. They should not be taken as evidence of complex focal seizures, which require entirely different management (Table 3.3).

Prognosis

*For myself I shall be well satisfied if I have made it appear proba-
ble to you that there does exist a form of epilepsy in children which
is distinguishable by its clinical features and in which the prognosis is always good.*

Adie[62] on pyknolepsy (CAE)

By applying strict criteria for diagnosis, the prognosis of CAE is excellent,[54,61,70] as Adie had found.[55] Remission occurs before the age of 12 years.
Less than 10% of the patients may develop infrequent or solitary GTCSs in
adolescence or adult life. It is exceptional for patients to continue having
absence seizures in their adult life.

Poor social adjustment of patients with CAE has been reported.[61] A more
recent report[71] found that of 69 children diagnosed but not necessarily suffering
from genuine CAE, 25% of had subtle cognitive deficits, 43% linguistic difficulties,
61% a psychiatric diagnosis, particularly attention deficit hyperactivity disorder
and anxiety disorders, and 30% clinically relevant attention and somatic com-
plaints, followed by social and thought problems. Duration of illness, seizure
frequency, and AED treatment were related to the severity of the cognitive, linguistic, and psychiatric comorbidities.[71] The same authors in another report
found that brain MRI showed significantly smaller grey matter volumes of the
left orbital frontal gyrus as well as both left and right temporal lobes compared
to children without epilepsy.[72] Male gender and an earlier age of diagnosis may
be associated with the need for two medications for seizure control in CAE.[73]

Management[54,74,75]

Monotherapy with either valproate or ethosuximide controls absences in
80% of patients.[75] Another option is lamotrigine monotherapy, although this
is less effective with around half of patients becoming seizure free.[75-77]

If monotherapy fails or unacceptable adverse reactions appear, the used
drug should be replaced by another. Adding small doses of lamotrigine to
valproate may be the best combination in resistant cases.

There are anecdotal reports that children may not respond to syrup of valproate despite adequate levels, but seizures stop if this is replaced with tablets
of valproate.[75] Sometimes seizures stop only with maximum tolerated doses of
valproate. It is my experience that once seizure cessation has been achieved,
valproate may be safely reduced to more moderate doses without relapses.[75]

Contraindicated drugs, either because they are ineffective or make seizures
worse, are carbamazepine, gabapentin, oxcarbazepine, phenytoin, phenobarbital, pregabalin, tiagabine and vigabatrin.

Withdrawing anti-epileptic medication: in the pure form of CAE, drug
therapy can be gradually withdrawn (over 3–6 months) after 2 or 3 years free
of seizures.

Epilepsy with Myoclonic Absences

Epilepsy with myoclonic absences (MAE)[78-82] is a rare IGE syndrome of childhood that demands scrupulous exclusion of other forms of symptomatic and cryptogenic cases manifesting with the same seizure (myoclonic absences).

Cosiderations on Classification

Myoclonic absences (the seizures) may feature either in normal or neurologically and mentally abnormal children.[61,80-82] MAE was previously categorised among the 'cryptogenic or symptomatic generalised epilepsies and syndromes'.[21] The new ILAE diagnostic scheme considers only the idiopathic form (Table 1.1),[25] which probably represents less than a third of the whole spectrum of epileptic disorders manifesting with myoclonic absences. The others are symptomatic or probably symptomatic cases.[21]

Demographic Data

Onset varies from the first months of life to the early teens (peak 7 years). Boys predominate. MAE is very rare. I have seen only three cases over a period of 15 years out of nearly 200 patients with video-EEG-recorded TAS.[22,23]

Clinical Manifestations

The myoclonic absences are the defining symptom of MAE (Fig. 4.1). These manifest with impairment of consciousness, which varies from mild to severe, and rhythmic myoclonic jerks, mainly of the shoulders, arms and legs, with a concomitant tonic contraction. Eyelid twitching is practically absent but perioral myoclonias are frequent. The jerks and the tonic contraction may be unilateral or asymmetrical and head/body unilateral deviation may be a constant feature in some patients. The tonic contraction mainly affects shoulder and deltoid muscles that may cause elevation of the arms. The duration of the absences varies from 8 to 60 s. Myoclonic absences occur many times per day.

C.P. Panayiotopoulos, *Idiopathic Generalised Epilepsies*,
DOI 10.1007/978-1-4471-4039-9_4, © Springer-Verlag London 2012

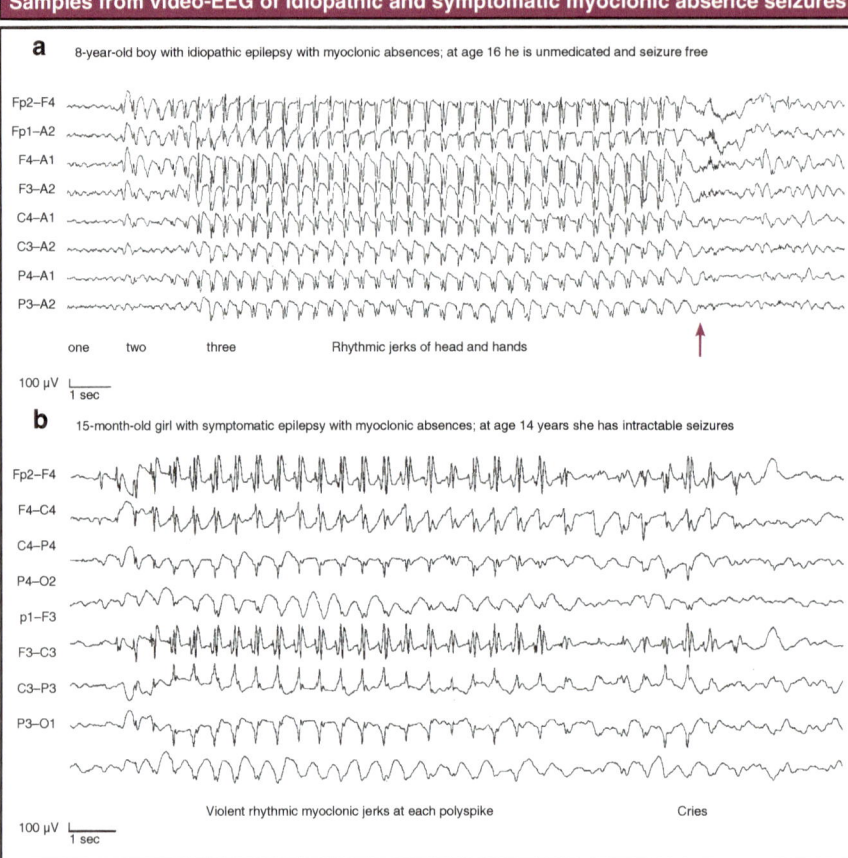

Fig. 4.1 (**a**) A video-EEG of a normal boy aged 8 years with myoclonic absences from age 6. The illustrated absence occurred during hyperventilation with breath counting (annotated) and it was terminated with somatosensory stimuli by tapping his shoulder (*red arrow*). Myoclonic absences were frequent, hundreds per day, and manifested with rhythmic myoclonic jerks and unresponsiveness. Valproate failed to achieve control, but absences ceased completely when ethosuximide was added to valproate at age 8. Medication was withdrawn at age 11. No further seizures occurred in the next 8 years of follow-up and he is academically successful. (**b**) Girl aged 15 months with myoclonic absences due to birth anoxia. Typical absence seizures started at 15 months of age. These were many per day, lasted for 8–10 s and were characterised by synchronous and bilateral myoclonic jerks of limbs and head with apparent loss of consciousness. Subsequently, she developed frequent, mainly nocturnal GTCSs, while myoclonic absences continued. These were intractable to any appropriate medication. At age 14 years she has significant learning difficulties, spastic paraparesis and numerous epileptic seizures. See video-EEG of these cases in the companion CD of *The Epilepsies: Seizures, Syndromes and Management*[23]

Absence status epilepticus is rare.

Other seizures, such as GTCSs or atonic fits, occur in two-thirds of patients, often predicting an unfavourable prognosis (these are probably symptomatic cases).

Aetiology

Myoclonic absences (the seizures, not the syndrome) are due to idiopathic, cryptogenic or symptomatic causes including chromosomal abnormalities.[83] A third are idiopathic and only these belong to this syndrome.

Diagnostic Procedures

By definition, in MAE all other tests but EEG should be normal. Brain MRI and chromosomal testing[83] are needed for the detection of symptomatic cases.

Electroencephalography

Background EEG is usually normal at onset but may deteriorate or be abnormal in symptomatic cases. In half of cases, inter-ictal EEG shows brief, generalised, focal or multifocal spike and slow wave.

Ictal EEG shows rhythmic 3 Hz GPSWD even in those with unilateral or asymmetrical clinical manifestations (Fig. 4.1). Polygraphic studies have revealed that each myoclonic jerk coincides with the spike component of the discharge.[80,82]

Differential Diagnosis

The differential diagnosis of MAE from other syndromes with absences is easy because of the characteristic type of myoclonic absences. The difficulty is between idiopathic and symptomatic/cryptogenic cases that manifest with the same seizure type (myoclonic absences). Symptomatic cases often have an abnormal neurological state, abnormal background EEG and abnormal brain MRI. Chromosomal abnormalities are common.[83] Additionally, absences with rhythmic myoclonic jerking but less than 2.5 Hz GPSWD and other characteristics of atypical absences may occur in epileptic encephalopathies,[84,85] and these may account for some of the cases with chromosomal abnormalities.[83]

Prognosis

Nearly half of children with MAE have impaired cognitive functioning prior to the onset of absences, but these are probably symptomatic cases. However, half of those who were normal prior to the onset of absences develop cognitive and behavioural impairment. This may mean a deteriorating effect of the EEG discharges on cognition.

Management

Myoclonic absences are often resistant to treatment. Half of patients (probably the symptomatic ones) continue having seizures in adult life, developing features of other types of epilepsy such as Lennox–Gastaut syndrome or JME.

Early control of absences may prevent subsequent cognitive deterioration and secure normal development. Treatment frequently requires high doses of valproate often combined with ethosuximide or small doses of lamotrigine. Clonazepam and acetazolamide may be used in polytherapy.

Juvenile Absence Epilepsy

Juvenile absence epilepsy (JAE) is an IGE syndrome[21,25,86] mainly manifesting with severe TAS. Nearly all patients (80%) also suffer from GTCSs and a fifth from sporadic myoclonic jerks.[22,23,87,88]

Considerations on Classification

The ILAE Task Force has not yet reached definite conclusions regarding the definition of JAE, although there is a tendency to consider JAE as part of a broader syndrome of IGE in adolescence.[20,25]

The 1989 ILAE classification broadly defined JAE by frequency of absences (less frequent than of CAE) and age at onset (around puberty).[21] These are insufficient criteria for the categorisation of any syndrome.[74] Thus, epidemiology, genetics, age at onset, clinical manifestations, other types of seizure, long-term prognosis and treatment may not accurately reflect the syndrome of JAE. JAE can be accurately defined on a cluster of video-EEG-studied clinical and EEG manifestations (Table 5.1).[22,86]

Inclusion criteria for JAE

Unequivocal clinical evidence of absence seizures with severe impairment of consciousness. Nearly all patients may have GTCSs. A fifth have myoclonic jerks, but these are mild and do not show the circadian distribution of JME

Documentation of ictal 3–4 Hz GPSWD, >4 s, that are associated with severe impairment of consciousness and often with automatisms. Normal EEG in treated patients are common

Exclusion criteria for JAE

The following may be incompatible with JAE

Clinical exclusion criteria:

Absences with marked eyelid or perioral myoclonus or marked single or rhythmic limb and trunk myoclonic jerks

Absences with exclusively mild or clinically undetectable impairment of consciousness

Consistent visual, photosensitive and other sensory precipitation of clinical absences is probably against the diagnosis of JAE. However, on the EEG, intermittent photic stimulation often facilitates generalised discharges and absences

EEG exclusion criteria:

Irregular, arrhythmic GPSWD with marked variations of the intradischarge frequency

Significant variations between the spike/polyspike and slow wave relations in GPSWD

Predominantly brief discharges (<4 s)

Table 5.1 Main inclusion and exclusion criteria for JAE

Demographic Data

Peak age at onset is 9–13 years (70% of patients) but range is from 5 to 20 years.[86,88] Myoclonic jerks and GTCSs usually begin 1–10 years after the onset of absences. Rarely, GTCSs may precede the onset of absences.[86,87] Both sexes are equally affected. Exact prevalence of JAE is not known because of variable criteria. In adults older than 20 years, prevalence of JAE may be around 2% or 3% of all epilepsies and around 8–10% of IGE.[89,90]

Clinical Manifestations

Frequent and severe typical absences are the characteristic and defining seizures of JAE (Fig. 5.1). The usual frequency of absences is approximately one to ten per day but this may be much higher for some patients.[86-88] Nearly all patients also develop GTCSs and a fifth of them also suffer from mild myoclonic jerks.

Typical absences are severe and frequent, often daily, and very similar to those of CAE, although they may be milder. The hallmark of the absence is abrupt, brief and severe impairment of consciousness with total or partial unresponsiveness. Mild or inconspicuous impairment of consciousness is not compatible with JAE. The ongoing voluntary activity usually stops at onset but may be partly restored during the ictus. Automatisms are frequent, usually occurring 6–10 s after the onset of the EEG discharge (Fig. 6.1). In JAE, mild myoclonic elements of the eyelids are common during the absence.

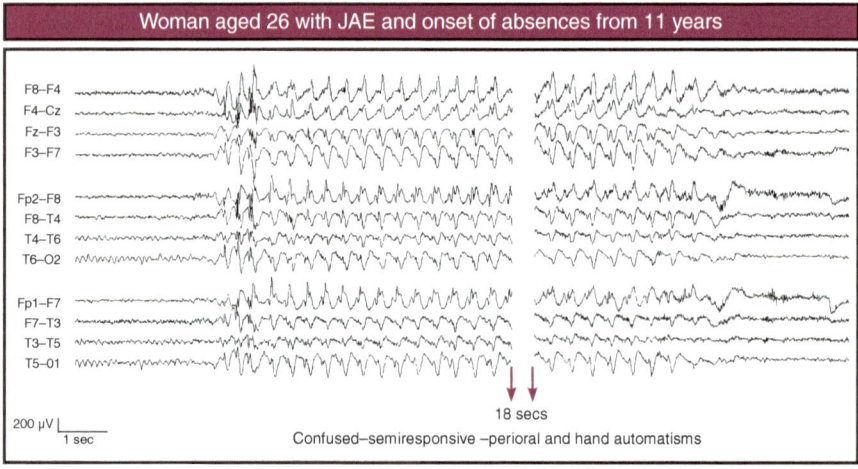

Fig. 5.1 From video-EEG of a 26-year-old normal woman. She started having frequent (tens per day) typical absence seizures with severe impairment of consciousness at age 11 years. At age 14 years she had her first GTCS. Since then, long absences of 20–30 s continue daily. Also she has three to five GTCSs every year, mainly in the morning after awakening. These are preceded by clusters of absences. Occasionally, she also has random, infrequent and mild limb myoclonic jerks, which started at age 20. Treatment with various appropriate anti-absence drugs resulted in minor improvement, but compliance varies

However, more severe and sustained myoclonic jerks of facial muscles may indicate another IGE with absences. Severe eyelid or perioral myoclonus, rhythmic limb jerking and single or arrhythmic myoclonic jerks of the head, trunk or limbs during the absence ictus are probably incompatible with JAE.

Duration of the absences varies from 4 to 30 s but it is usually long (about 16 s).

GTCSs are probably unavoidable in untreated patients. GTCSs occur in 80% of patients, mainly after awakening, although nocturnal or diurnal GTCSs may also be experienced.[86-89,91,92] GTCSs are usually infrequent but they may also become severe and intractable.

Myoclonic jerks occurring in 15–25% of the patients are infrequent, mild and of random distribution. They usually occur in the afternoon hours when the patient is tired, rather than in the morning after awakening.[86,93]

Absence status epilepticus is truly generalised non-convulsive (without any type of jerks or convulsions) and occurs in a fifth of patients.[94]

Seizure-Precipitating Factors

Mental and psychological arousal is the main precipitating factor for typical absences. Conversely, sleep deprivation, fatigue, alcohol, excitement and lights, alone or usually in combination, are the main precipitating factors for GTCSs.

Some authors reported that 8% of JAE patients suffered from photosensitivity clinically or on EEG.[87] However, clinical photosensitivity, which is a consistent provocation of seizures (absences, GTCSs or jerks), may be incompatible with JAE. These patients may belong to other IGEs.[86] EEG photosensitivity that is facilitation of absences by IPS may not be uncommon.

Aetiology

JAE is determined by genetic factors but its mode of transmission and relation to other forms of IGE, particularly CAE and JME, has not yet been established; a single Mendelian mode appears to be unlikely.

There is an increased incidence of epileptic disorders in families of patients with JAE and there are reports of monozygotic twins with JAE.[22,88,95] A proband with JAE was found in three of 37 families selected because at least three members were affected by IGE in one or more generations.[96] However, only one sibling also had JAE, while other members mainly had GTCSs.[96]

JAE may be linked to chromosome 8,[97] 21,[98] 18[99] and probably 5.[99] Heterogeneity may be common. Autopsy[100] and MRI studies[101] found microdysgenesis and other cerebral microstructural changes in patients with JAE.

Diagnostic Procedures

All but EEG tests are normal.

Electroencephalography

The EEG in untreated patients is abnormal with absences easily elicited by hyperventilation (Fig. 5.1). The background inter-ictal EEG is normal. Focal epileptiform abnormalities and abortive asymmetrical bursts of spikes/ polyspikes are common.

The ictal EEG shows 3–4 Hz GPSWD. The frequency at the initial phase of the discharge is usually fast (3–5 Hz). There is a gradual and smooth decline in frequency from the initial to the terminal phase. The discharge is regular, with well-formed spikes and polyspikes, which retain a constant relation with the slow waves (Fig. 5.1).

Differential Diagnosis

In general, and particularly in adults, absences are often misdiagnosed as complex focal seizures, although their differentiation is easy.[102]

The differentiation of JAE from other IGEs with absences may be more difficult without appropriate video-EEG evaluation.[22,86] In children, it is often difficult to distinguish between CAE and JAE, because their features overlap and manifestations are similar. In JAE absences often start at a later age, usually they are less frequent and impairment of cognition is less severe.[22] Automatisms are equally prominent in both. Limb myoclonic jerks (not during the absences) and/or GTCSs in the presence of severe absences indicate JAE.

JAE is distinctly different from Jeavons syndrome of very brief seizures marked with rapid eyelid myoclonia, perioral myoclonia with absences (PMA) of rhythmic perioral myoclonia during the absence, and MAE of rhythmic myoclonic jerks.

In adolescents, the differential diagnosis should not be difficult between JAE and JME (Table 5.2). Severe absences are the major problem in JAE;

	JME	JAE
Main type of seizures	Myoclonic jerks	Typical absences
Circadian distribution	Mainly on awakening	Any time during the day
Typical absences	Mild and often imperceptible; they occur in a third of patients	Defining seizure type; they are very severe and occur in all patients
Myoclonic jerks	Defining seizure type; they occur in all patients and mainly on awakening	Mild; they occur in a fifth of patients and are random
GTCS	They mainly occur after a series of myoclonic jerks on awakening	They mainly occur independently or less commonly after a series of absence seizures
EEG	Brief (1–3 s) 3–6 Hz GPSWD, which are usually asymptomatic	Lengthy (8–30 s) 3–4 Hz GPSWD, which are usually associated with severe impairment of consciousness

Table 5.2 Key differences between JME and JAE

myoclonic jerks are the main seizure type in JME. Absences in JME are mild and often inconspicuous.

Prognosis

JAE is a lifelong disorder although seizures can be controlled in 70–80% of patients. However, there is a tendency for the absences to become less severe in terms of impairment of cognition, duration and frequency with age and particularly after the fourth decade of life. GTCSs are usually infrequent, often precipitated by sleep deprivation, fatigue and alcohol consumption. Myoclonic jerks, if present, are not troublesome for the patient. A fifth of the patients have frequent and sometimes intractable absences and GTCSs, and this figure may be higher if appropriate treatment is not initiated at early stages of JAE.

Management

The treatment of IGE is detailed from page 61. In JAE, the consensus is that, because of the frequent combination of absences and GTCSs, the drug of choice is valproate, which controls all seizure types in 70–80% of the JAE patients. Lamotrigine, which controls absence seizures and GTCSs in around 50–60% of patients, is probably another good monotherapy option in cases, for example in women, where valproate is unsuitable.

If monotherapy with valproate is partially effective, add-on treatment with small doses of lamotrigine (particularly if GTCS is the problem) or ethosuximide (particularly if absences persist) may further improve or control the situation.

Control of absences is usually (90%) associated with good control of GTCSs and it is adversely affected by the frequency and the duration of GTCSs before starting valproate treatment.

Levetiracetam is formally indicated for GTCS and myoclonic jerks of IGEs as documented with RCTs.[103,104] Recent evidence suggests that levetiracetam is also effective in absences seizures of IGEs including juvenile absence epilepsy.[105-108]

The role of other newer drugs such as topiramate and zonisamide has not been properly evaluated.

Patients should be warned regarding precipitating factors of GTCS.

Treatment may be lifelong because attempts to withdraw medication nearly invariably leads to relapses, even after many years free of seizures.

Juvenile Myoclonic Epilepsy

Synonym: JME, Janz syndrome.

This syndrome is one of the most important IGEs that is genetically determined.[109-113] The frequent errors in its diagnosis and management are avoidable.

Demographic Data

The triad of absences, jerks and GTCSs shows a characteristic age-related onset. Absences, when a feature, begin between the ages of 5 and 16 years. Myoclonic jerks follow 1–9 years later, usually about the age of 14 or 15 years. GTCSs normally appear a few months later than the myoclonic jerks, although they can occasionally appear earlier. Both sexes are equally affected. Prevalence is 8–10% among adult and adolescent patients with epilepsies.[1,23,112]

Clinical Manifestations

JME is characterised by:
- Myoclonic jerks on awakening
- GTCSs in nearly all patients
- Typical absences in more than a third of the patients.

> *Lots of blanks and jerks; then I had a grand mal… I usually have fits when rushing after getting up; usually does not happen later in the day.*[109]

Myoclonic jerks occurring after awakening are the most prominent and characteristic seizure type.[11,112,114-117] They are shock-like, irregular and arrhythmic clonic movements of proximal and distal muscles mainly of the upper extremities. They are often inconspicuous, restricted to the fingers, making the patient prone to drop things or look clumsy. They may be violent enough to cause falls. A fifth of patients describe their jerks as unilateral, but video-EEG shows that the jerks affect both sides (Fig. 6.1).[115,117]

Some patients (<10%) with mild forms of JME never develop GTCSs.[112]

Typical absence seizures: A third of patients have typical absences, which are brief with subtle impairment of consciousness (Figs. 6.2 and 6.3). They are different from the absence seizures of CAE or JAE.[22,114,118]

C.P. Panayiotopoulos, *Idiopathic Generalised Epilepsies*,
DOI 10.1007/978-1-4471-4039-9_6, © Springer-Verlag London 2012

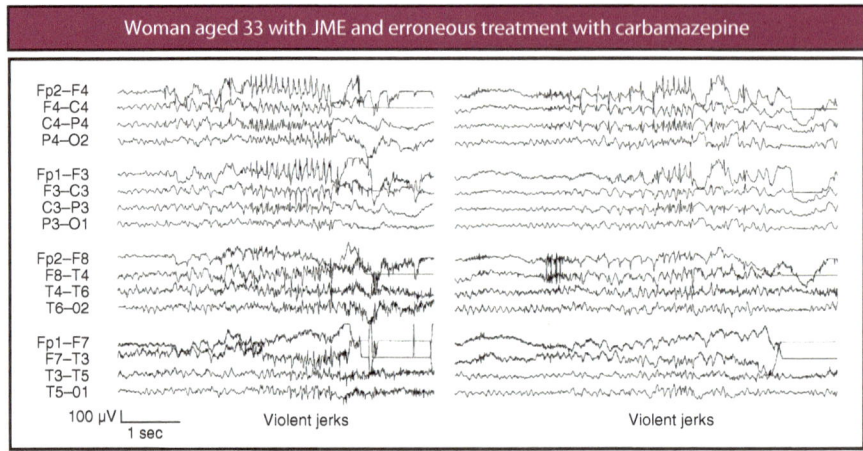

Fig. 6.1 Samples from the video-EEG of a woman with JME but on erroneous AED treatment with carbamazepine. Violent myoclonic jerks occur with generalised polyspike discharges (see also Fig. 6.4 of the same patient)

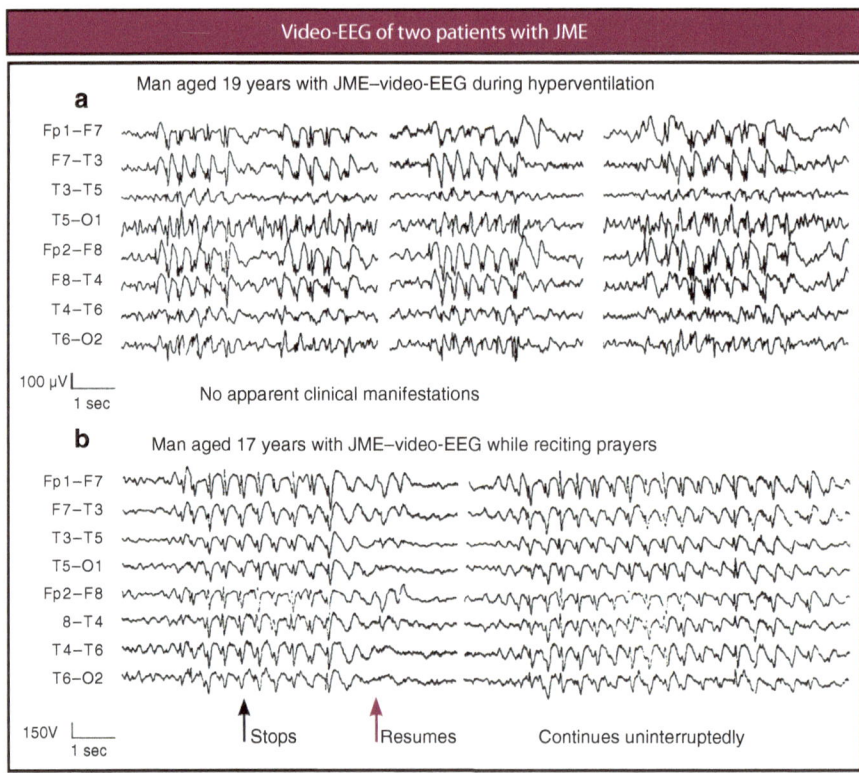

Fig. 6.2 (**a**) GPSWD are not associated with apparent clinical manifestations (but these may have been revealed if breath counting was performed during hyperventilation). (**b**) GPSWD are associated with mild impairment of cognition (Modified with permission from Panayiotopoulos et al.[22])

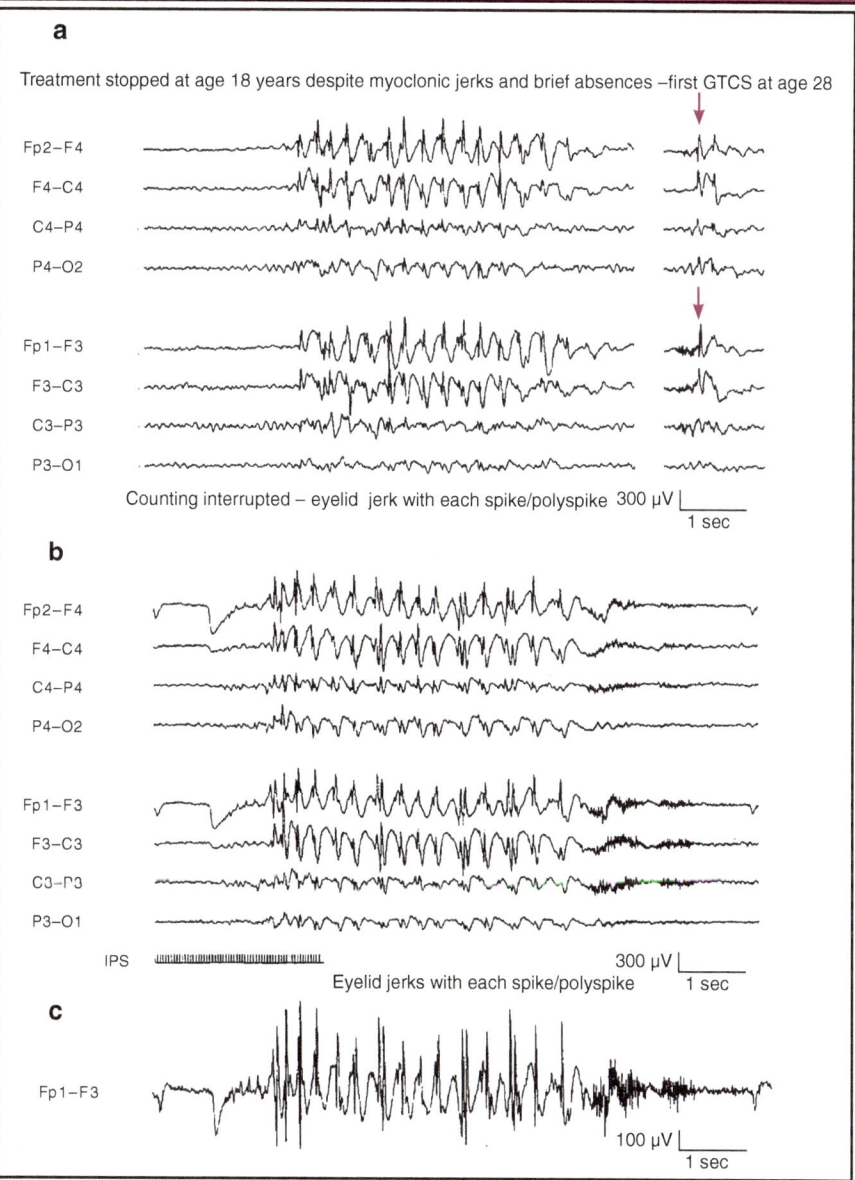

Sample from a video-EEG of a woman, aged 28 years, who had suffered from JME since the age of 9 years

a

Treatment stopped at age 18 years despite myoclonic jerks and brief absences –first GTCS at age 28

Fp2–F4
F4–C4
C4–P4
P4–O2

Fp1–F3
F3–C3
C3–P3
P3–O1

Counting interrupted – eyelid jerk with each spike/polyspike   300 µV
1 sec

b

Fp2–F4
F4–C4
C4–P4
P4–O2

Fp1–F3
F3–C3
C3–P3
P3–O1

IPS   300 µV
Eyelid jerks with each spike/polyspike   1 sec

c

Fp1–F3

100 µV
1 sec

Fig. 6.3 This woman was referred for a routine EEG because she had experienced 'probable IGE-absences from age 9 until age 18 years. Myoclonus as a teenager when sleep deprived. Recently suffered her first ever GTCS following sleep deprivation. No absence or myoclonus for 10 years. Treatment with valproate was withdrawn at age 18 years.' The video-EEG documented that she still had brief absences, which manifest with mild impairment of cognition and eyelid jerks. These were spontaneous, or induced by (**a**) hyperventilation and (**b**) intermittent photic stimulation. Note the polyspike wave of the discharges and the irregular intradischarge frequency (**c**). Also note the bifrontal spike-slow wave discharges (**a**, *red arrows*)

Absences appearing before the age of 10 years may be more severe. They become less frequent and severe with age.[22,114,118]

A tenth of patients do not perceive absences, despite GPSWD lasting for more than 3 s.[112,118] However, on video-EEG with breath counting during hyperventilation, such EEG discharges often manifest with mild impairment of cognition, eyelid flickering or both (Figs. 6.2 and 6.3).[75]

GTCSs usually follow the onset of myoclonic jerks.[111,112,114-116,119]

Myoclonic jerks, usually in clusters and often with an accelerating frequency and severity, may precede a GTCS, a so-called clonic–tonic–clonic generalised seizure.[115]

Status epilepticus: Myoclonic status epilepticus is probably more common than appreciated.[112,120] This almost invariably starts on awakening, often precipitated by sleep deprivation, or missing medication. Consciousness may not be impaired, although in some patients absences are often interspersed with myoclonic jerks (Fig. 6.4).

Pure absence status epilepticus[94] is very rare. Generalised tonic–clonic status epilepticus is infrequent. For further details on status epilepticus.

Circadian distribution: Seizures, principally myoclonic jerks, occur within 30 min–1 h of awakening. Myoclonic jerks rarely occur at other times unless

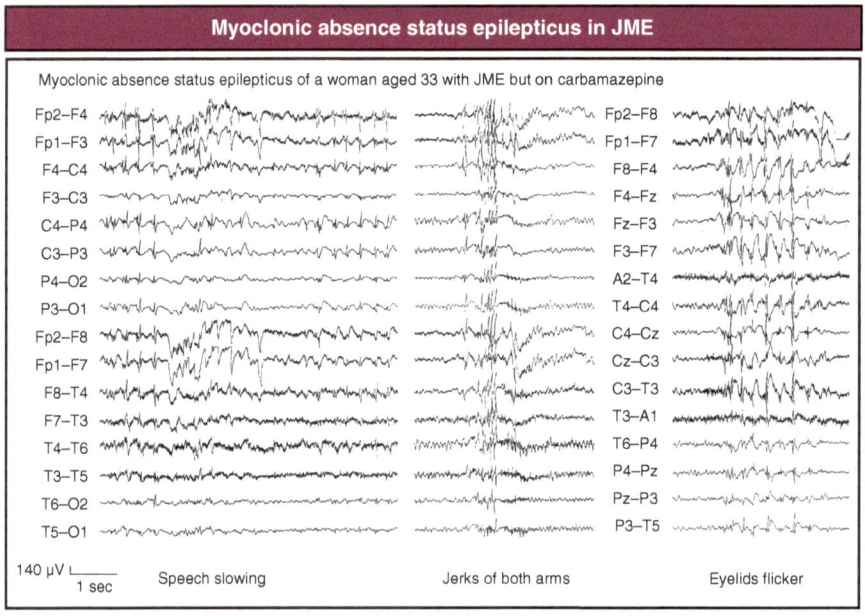

Myoclonic absence status epilepticus in JME

Myoclonic absence status epilepticus of a woman aged 33 with JME but on carbamazepine

140 μV | 1 sec   Speech slowing   Jerks of both arms   Eyelids flicker

Fig. 6.4 Video-EEG of a woman with classical JME, but on carbamazepine at the time of this recording (see also Fig. 6.1 from the same patient). The patient was mildly confused with continuous jerking of the hands (middle) and, rarely, the eyelids. The ictal EEG consisted of repetitive and discontinuous frequent GPSWD interrupted by brief intervals of relative normality. Each GPSWD consisted of varying numbers of polyspikes/spikes–wave in various combinations and morphologies

the patient is tired. GTCSs occur mainly on awakening preceded by clusters of myoclonic jerks, but may also be purely nocturnal or random. Absence seizures rarely show a circadian predilection.

Seizure-Precipitating Factors

Sleep deprivation and fatigue, particularly after excessive alcohol intake, are the most powerful precipitants of jerks and GTCSs in JME.

> ### Useful Note
>
> Sleep deprivation means a late night followed by a brief sleep suddenly interrupted by either compulsory early awakening in order to go to work or on a trip. An unscheduled telephone call early next morning may frequently have disastrous effects.

Photosensitivity is confirmed with EEG in more than 30% of patients but this may be of no clinical significance. Probably less than a tenth of patients have seizures induced by photic stimulation in daily life (Fig. 6.3).

Other common and prominent seizure-precipitating factors include mental stress and emotions, in particular excitement, concentration, mental and psychological arousal, failed expectations or frustration.

Personality, behavioural, cognitive and psychological aberrations have been frequently reported in patients with JME.[114,121-124]

Aetiology

JME is a genetically determined syndrome.[2,111,119,125] Around 50–60% of families of probands with JME report seizures in first- or second-degree relatives.[119,126] Inheritance is probably complex.[127-129] The proposed models of inheritance include polygenic with a lower manifestation threshold for females, autosomal dominant with variable penetrance, a two-locus model with a dominant gene on chromosome 6p and an as-yet-unknown recessive gene, or the possibility that different genotypes with different modes of inheritance underlie the phenotype.[130]

Families with autosomal[125] or dominant[125,127] mendelian inheritance have been described, but these may be rare.

Molecular studies favour a susceptibility locus for JME in chromosome 6p11–12 (*EJM1*)[129] or 15q14 (*EJM2*).[131,132] A gene, *C6orf33*, in the *EJM1* region has been identified.[133] An association of JME with an HLA-DR allele[134,135] was not replicated.[136]

Genetic heterogeneity of JME is a possible explanation for such discordant observations.

It has been hypothesised that JME is a frontal lobe variant of a multiregional, thalamocortical network epilepsy rather than a generalised epilepsy syndrome.[137]

Diagnostic Procedures

All tests except EEG are normal. Using new MRI technologies, abnormalities involving mesio-frontal cortical structures have been reported in some patients with JME.[123,138]

Electroencephalography

The EEG in untreated patients is usually abnormal, with 3–6 Hz GPSWD, and with intradischarge fragmentations and unstable intradischarge frequency (Figs. 6.2 and 6.3). A third of the patients show photoparoxysmal responses. A third may also have focal EEG abnormalities of single spikes, spike–wave complexes or slow waves.[22]

A normal EEG in a patient suspected of having JME should prompt an EEG during sleep and awakening.

The typical EEG discharge of a myoclonic jerk is a generalised burst of polyspikes of 0.5–2 s duration (Figs. 6.1 and 6.4).

The ictal discharges of absences in JME are distinctly different from those in CAE and JAE.[22,118] They consist of spike/double/treble or polyspikes usually preceding or superimposed on the slow waves (Figs. 6.2, 6.3, 6.4 and 6.5). Polyspikes consist of up to eight to ten spikes with a characteristic 'worm-like' or compressed capital W appearance ('Ws'). The number and amplitude of spikes shows considerable inter- and intradischarge variation. The intradischarge frequency of the GPSWD varies from 2 to 10 Hz, with a mean of 3–5 Hz. The frequency is often higher in the first second from onset. Fragmentations of the discharge are common and characteristic. Ws and fragmentation of discharges are observed in all patients, but vary quantitatively between patients and between discharges (Figs. 6.2 and 6.3).

Brief discharges are far more common than long ones, and most of the discharges last for 1–4 s.

Differential Diagnosis

JME is a typical example of a frequently misdiagnosed common epileptic syndrome resulting in avoidable morbidity.[139,140] Failure to diagnose JME is a serious medical error because JME defies all aspects of general advice regarding 'epilepsy'. Diagnosis should improve with heightened medical awareness. Physicians should be ever alert to the possibility of JME.

The rate of misdiagnosis of JME is as high as 90%.[139,140] Factors responsible include lack of familiarity with JME, failure to elicit a history of myoclonic jerks, misinterpretation of absences as complex focal seizures, misinterpretation of jerks as focal motor seizures, and high prevalence of focal EEG abnormalities.

JME is easy to diagnose because of a characteristic clustering of myoclonic and other generalised seizures of IGEs, circadian distribution, precipitating factors and EEG manifestations. Patients are otherwise normal and there is no mental or physical deterioration if properly diagnosed and treated.

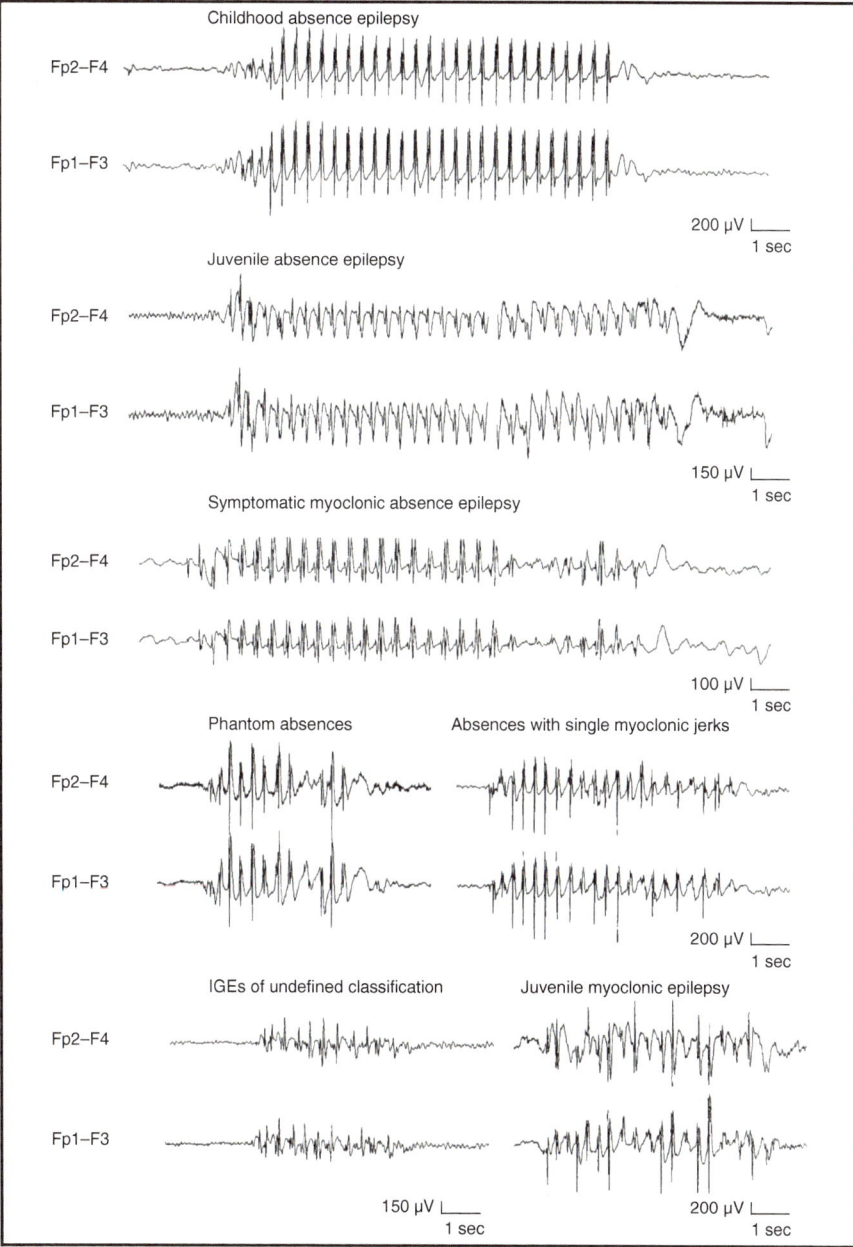

Fig. 6.5 These seven patients had different syndromes of idiopathic and symptomatic absence epilepsies. Note that the GSWD may be brief or prolonged, with or without polyspikes and of regular or irregular sequence. Also, note that the intradischarge frequency of the spike–wave complexes may show marked diversity. Although there are significant variations between different syndromes, the GSWD is not itself pathognomonic of any syndrome. The syndromic diagnosis requires homogenous clustering of symptoms and signs

Of other IGEs, JAE may be more difficult to differentiate because this syndrome may also manifest with similar clinical and EEG manifestations. The main differentiating factor is that absences with severe impairment of consciousness, not the myoclonic jerks, are the main seizure type in JAE (Table 13.5). Myoclonic jerks, if they occur, are mild and random often lacking the circadian distribution of JME.

Another formidable situation is when JME starts with absences in childhood prior to the development of myoclonic jerks. There are no prospective video-EEG studies of these patients. Retrospectively examining EEG and clinical manifestations of these patients, I am of the opinion that their absences are distinct from CAE or JAE in that they are usually shorter and milder, and ictal EEG often contains GPSWD. Certainly, this situation is not CAE progressing to JME as some authors reported.[141] It is JME starting with absences prior to the development of myoclonic jerks.

Diagnostic Tips

GTCSs, usually preceded by myoclonic jerks, are nearly pathognomonic of JME if they occur in the morning after:

- A party to celebrate, for example, a birthday, the end of school term or New Year's eve
- Waking up early in the morning to travel for vacations, particularly after a late night
- Replacement of valproate with carbamazepine in women wishing to start a family
- Withdrawal of appropriate medication after many seizure-free years.

Diagnostic Tips

Revealing myoclonic jerks is an essential part of diagnosing JME

Elicitation of the characteristic history of myoclonic jerks is something of an art. It is often necessary to physically demonstrate mild myoclonic jerks of the fingers and hands, and to inquire about morning clumsiness and tremors.[142] Questions like 'do you spill your morning tea?' and 'do you drop things in the morning?', together with a simultaneous demonstration of how myoclonic jerks produce this effect, may be answered positively by patients who denied experiencing myoclonic jerks on direct questioning. Further elaboration is required to confirm that clumsiness was due to genuine myoclonic jerks. If the patient reports normal hypnagogic jactitations, it is reassuring that the concept of myoclonic jerks has been understood. Diagnostic yield may be improved by emphasising the close relationship between jerks and fatigue, alcohol and sleep deprivation. Some patients do not report their jerks, erroneously assuming that this is a self-inflicted normal phenomenon related to excess of alcohol and lack of sleep.

Prognosis

All seizures are probably lifelong, although improving after the fourth decade of life.[143] JME may vary in severity from mild myoclonic jerks to frequent and severe falls and GTCSs if not appropriately diagnosed and treated.

Seizures are generally well controlled with appropriate medication in up to 90% of patients.[109,112,115,144] Patients with all three types of seizure are more likely to be resistant to treatment.[145]

Management

Advice regarding life-style, avoidance of precipitating factors and long-term medication is essential for a patient with an incontrovertible diagnosis of JME. Avoidance of alcohol indulgence and compensating for sleep deprivation is mandatory. Some patients with mild forms of JME have GTCSs or myoclonic jerks only after excessively violating these factors.

Pharmacological Treatment

All formal current recommendations discourage or practically prohibit the use of valproate in women of childbearing age but provide no documented alternatives for their treatment in JME, where valproate has been the first line AED for the last 30 years.

> *Converging evidence from multiple and independent sources indicate that levetiracetam is the first choice AED in the treatment in at least women with JME.*

Valproate is the most effective AED in the treatment of JME, but is humbled by serious adverse reactions in women and has not been yet compared with levetiracetam in face to face RCTs. However, it may still be considered as first line AED therapy in men with JME.

Levetiracetam is the likely candidate to replace valproate in the treatment of JME:

(a) In non-control independent studies, 62–67% of patients with intractable JME, including those that have failed with valproate, became seizure free with levetiracetam monotherapy or polytherapy. This high rate of response to levetiracetam has been confirmed in recent more systematic studies of monotherapy[146] or conversion to monotherapy from polytherapy (including valproate failures).[147]

(b) Levetiracetam is the first and only newer AED licensed for the treatment of myoclonic seizures in JME (adjunctive therapy in adults and adolescents) because of its efficacy and safety tested in RCT.[148]

(c) It appears to have a favourable profile in women and pregnancy.

(d) It has high and sustained efficacy, fast action, good safety profile, and lack of clinically meaningful interactions with other drugs.[12,149]

Lamotrigine is widely used in JME because:

(a) It was the first of the newer AEDs that appeared to be effective in JME, but this was mainly in combination with valproate; its promyoclonic effect as monotherapy became apparent much later[150,151]

(b) It was promoted as the only alternative to valproate in women; its interactions with hormonal contraception and pregnancy that may lead to seizure deterioration or toxicity, as well as the uncertainties surrounding its teratogenic potential, only recently have been reported.[152-156]

Considering all this new information, compounded with the high rate of idiosyncratic ADRs, necessity for slow titration and drug-to-drug interactions, lamotrigine monotherapy in JME patients is questionable.

Clonazepam administered in small doses (0.5–2 mg at night) is probably the most effective treatment for myoclonic jerks. However, clonazepam alone may not suppress GTCSs.[112,157] Furthermore, clonazepam may deprive patients of the warning of an impending GTCS provided by the myoclonic jerks.[112,157] In mild JME with myoclonic jerks only, clonazepam alone may be recommended.

When cost is of concern, *phenobarbital* is the best option. It is effective in about 60% of patients.

Topiramate and *zonisamide* are by far second options, particularly in women.

Contraindicated drugs include vigabatrin, tiagabine, gabapentin, pregabalin, phenytoin, oxcarbazepine and carbamazepine. Carbamazepine is not effective in jerks and absences but it is possibly effective on GTCSs of IGEs.

See details of the treatment of IGEs in chapter 13.

Prevention of GTCSs and Termination of Myoclonic and Absence Status Epilepticus

It is important to remember that patients with JME often experience myoclonic jerks or myoclonic-absence status epilepticus long before terminating to a GTCS. This can be prevented by home administration of an appropriate benzodiazepine preparation and preferably buccal midazolam.

Duration of AED Treatment and Withdrawal of Medication

Lifelong treatment with proper AEDs is usually considered necessary in patients with JME. Withdrawal of appropriate medication results in relapses, even in patients who have been seizure free for many years with an appropriate AED.[112] In mild forms of JME, it may be safe to reduce the dose of medication slowly over months or years, especially after the fourth decade of life.[143] Persistence or recrudescence of myoclonic jerks necessitates continuation of medication.

Epilepsy with GTCS Only

GTCSs are a common feature in IGEs and occur predominantly on awakening. Overall, GTCSs are reported to occur on awakening (17–53% of patients), diffusely whilst awake (23–36%), during sleep (27–44%) or randomly (13–26%).[158] It is undetermined what proportion of these patients also has other generalised seizures (jerks or absences).

GTCSs are the most severe forms of epileptic seizures, while absences and myoclonic jerks may be mild and sometimes inconspicuous to the patient and imperceptible to the observer.[159,160] They are often detected only by meticulous history taking and video-EEG. A patient with a first GTCS has often suffered from minor seizures (absences, myoclonic jerks or both), sometimes many years prior to the GTCS.

Considerations on Classification

IGE with GTCS was only considered a syndrome in the new ILAE diagnostic scheme,[20,25] and incorporated 'epilepsy with GTCS on awakening (EGTCSA)' previously recognised as a separate syndrome.[21]

In the previous edition of this book, it was emphasised that 'IGE with GTCS only' has not been precisely defined by the ILAE Task Force.[25] Its name implies that it includes only those patients with GTCSs alone (i.e. without absences and/or jerks) and that these may occur at any time. However, it is more likely that it is a broader category (rather than a syndrome) of 'IGE with *predominantly* GTCS' (also including patients with mild absences, myoclonic jerks or both).

The new ILAE report[56] has now revised its position and specifies the following:

> *Epilepsy with GTCS only is not a syndrome, and the Core Group was unable to agree on any syndrome with this feature: the consistent diurnal pattern of seizures in some patients needs further investigation. Whether epilepsy with GTCS on awakening exists as a distinct entity is unclear.*

A genetically determined syndrome of 'intractable childhood epilepsy with GTCS' is probably unrelated to the 'epilepsy with GTCS only' covered in this chapter.

Demographic Data

Age at onset varies from 6 to 47 years with a peak at 16 or 17 years; 80% have their first GTCS in the second decade of life. Men (55%) slightly predominate over women, probably because of differences in alcohol exposure and sleep habits. The prevalence of IGE with GTCS only is unknown. In my studies with strict criteria (GTCS only)[23] this may be very small (0.9% of IGEs), but others have given a prevalence of 13–15% among IGEs.[161,162]

Clinical Manifestations

By definition all patients suffer from GTCSs but this syndrome has not been examined in its entirety. Only EGTCSA has been extensively studied[163-165] and is presented in this chapter.

Patients suffer from GTCSs, which occur within 1 or 2 h after awakening from either nocturnal or diurnal sleep. The seizure may occur while the patient is still in bed or having his breakfast or upon arriving at work. Seizures may also occur during relaxation or leisure.[158,163,164]

Janz described patients with EGTCSA as unreliable, unstable and prone to neglect.[164,165] The sleep patterns of EGTCSA patients are particularly unstable and modifiable by external factors (e.g. AEDs), and the patients may suffer from chronic sleep deficit.[158,163,164]

Seizure-Precipitating Factors

Sleep deprivation, fatigue and excessive alcohol consumption are the main seizure precipitants. Shift work, changes in sleep habits, particularly during holidays and celebrations, predispose to GTCSs on awakening. A quarter of patients are reported to show photosensitivity on EEG.[158]

Aetiology

There is a high incidence of epileptic disorders in families,[158,164] and a link to the *EJM1* locus has been reported.[166] Conversely, adolescent-onset idiopathic GTCS epilepsy with GTCS at any time, whilst awake, was not linked to the *EJM1* locus.[166] Severe IGE of infancy with GTCS is often related to mutations of the *SCN1A* gene.

Diagnostic Procedures

By definition all tests other than EEG are normal.

Electroencephalography

EEG shows GPSWD in half of patients with pure EGTCSA (Fig. 7.1) and 70% of those with additional absences or myoclonic jerks preceding GTCSs.

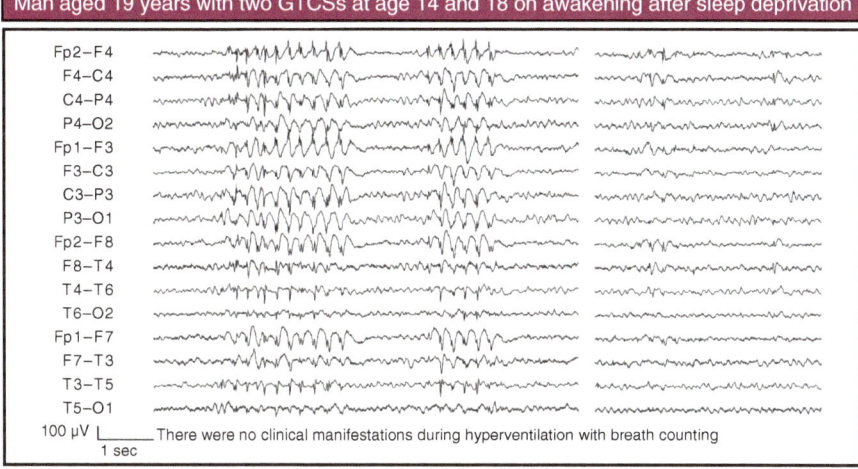

Fig. 7.1 Asymptomatic GPSWD on video-EEG of a 19-year-old university student who had two GTCSs at age 14 and 18. They both occurred half an hour after awakening from a brief sleep during exam periods. There was no clinical history of any other types of seizure and there were no other symptoms preceding either of the GTCSs. Note that the discharges may start from right or left. Also note focal spikes at various locations

A normal routine EEG should prompt a video-EEG performed on sleep and on awakening. Myoclonic jerks or, more frequently, brief absences will often be revealed. Focal EEG abnormalities in the absence of generalised discharges are rare. Photoparoxysmal responses are reported in 17% of females and 9% of males with EGTCSA.[158]

Differential Diagnosis

The differential diagnosis is mainly from patients with other IGEs, which share with EGTCSA the same propensity to seizures after awakening and the same precipitating factors. JME and JAE are examples of IGE syndromes, which may cause diagnostic difficulties. Rarely, secondarily GTCSs of focal epilepsies may also consistently occur on awakening.

Prognosis

As in all other types of IGE with onset in the mid-teens, EGTCSA is probably a lifelong disease with a high (83%) incidence of relapse on withdrawal of treatment.[158,163] Characteristically, the intervals between seizures become shorter with time, the precipitating factors less obvious, and GTCSs may become more random (diurnal and nocturnal), as a result of either the evolution of the disease or drug-induced modifications.

Management

Patients should be warned of the common seizure precipitants – sleep deprivation with early awaking and alcohol consumption – and when possible should avoid occupational night shifts. Patients, after adjusting their life styles, may become seizure free. Drug treatment is the same as for IGE with GTCSs.

Other Probable Syndromes of IGE to Consider

Implicitly, one must be prepared to split before one can lump. Thus we must always be on guard against unwittingly lumping because we are unaware of certain characteristics on which we should have split.

Berg and Blackstone[167]

Probable syndromes of IGE that are not officially recognised by the ILAE are[7,23,168]:

- IGE with absences of early childhood
- Perioral mycoclonia with absences
- IGE with phantom absences
- Monogenic IGE syndromes

Jeavons syndrome (eyelid myoclonia with absences), is described with the reflex epilepsies.

'Absence status epilepsy'[169] probably represent heterogeneous syndromes of IGE with absence status epilepticus, which is often the result of prior inappropriate AED treatment.

Video-EEG documentation of most of the syndromes described in this section can be found in the CD companion to references [23] and [26]. Their diagnosis in clinical practice is significant at least for genetic and prognostic reasons.

Significant Clinical Note

Of clinical importance is the diagnosis of absence seizures associated with GLUT1 deficiency syndrome. Seizures begin between age one and four months in 90% of cases. The frequency and severity of seizures varies among affected individuals. Typical or atypical absences, mainly of early onset are the most prominent seizure types. Typical absences may imitate various syndromes of idiopathic generalised epilepsy with absences such as epilepsy with myoclonic absences, childhood or juvenile absence epilepsy. The ketogenic diet is highly effective in controlling the seizures. An early diagnosis and early start of a ketogenic diet may prevent deterioration. Phenobarbital is contra-indicated.

Molecular genetic testing for SLC2A1, which is the only gene known to be associated with GLUT1 deficiency is now clinically available. Families with members manifesting various types of idiopathic generalized epilepsy with absences (early onset absence seizures, childhood or juvenile absence epilepsy, juvenile myoclonic epilepsy) should be tested for SLC2A1 gene mutations.[167a, 167b]

C.P. Panayiotopoulos, *Idiopathic Generalised Epilepsies*, DOI 10.1007/978-1-4471-4039-9_8, © Springer-Verlag London 2012

IGE with Absences of Early Childhood[91,170-173]

Typical absences starting from early childhood (a few months to 5 years of age) are not a specific expression of a distinct syndrome. This may be the first manifestation of MAE, perioral or eyelid myoclonia with absences, EM-AS, CAE or more severe forms of generalised epilepsies. By excluding all these, it is realistic to propose that there is a syndrome of IGE that starts in early childhood primarily manifesting with absences, often combined with GTCSs and possibly with myoclonic jerks.

Doose,[171,172] having studied 140 cases with onset of absences in early childhood, rightly concluded that 'this is an heterogeneous subgroup within IGE. There is a distinct overlap with early childhood epilepsy with GTCS and myoclonic–astatic epilepsy on the one side and with CAE on the other. Thus it should not be regarded as a special syndrome.'[171,172] I am in complete agreement with this statement. Age at onset of absence seizures alone cannot define an epileptic syndrome. However, with improved diagnostic skills, applying inclusion (e.g. including absences and GTCSs) and exclusion criteria (e.g. excluding CAE, EM-AS, MAE, PMA and possibly symptomatic cases) it appears there there is such an idiopathic generalised epilepsy that we have to define more precisely.

Based on currently available data, this is an IGE (occurring in otherwise normal children) with the following features:

- Absences are markedly different from CAE; clinically they are less severe and less frequent
- GTCSs are common (two-thirds) and often the first seizure type
- Myoclonic jerks and myoclonic–astatic seizures occur in 40%
- Absence status epilepticus is common and may lead to cognitive impairment
- Bboys are more likely to suffer GTCSs than girls
- Ictal EEG 3 or 4 Hz GPSWD is very irregular and termination is not abrupt but often fades with slow spike–wave
- Background EEG shows a moderate excess of slow waves
- Long-term prognosis is worse than in CAE
- Strong family history of IGE and GPSWD in EEG of unaffected members, particularly mothers.

C.P. Panayiotopoulos, *Idiopathic Generalised Epilepsies*,
DOI 10.1007/978-1-4471-4039-9_9, © Springer-Verlag London 2012

Perioral Myoclonia with Absences[174,175]

Typical absences with motor symptoms of perioral myoclonia is a non-specific symptom. However, this often combines with a clustering of other clinical and EEG features suggestive of an interesting syndrome of PMA within the IGEs.

Considerations on Classification

PMA has been recognised neither as a seizure type nor as a syndrome by the ILAE.[21,25] That absences with perioral myoclonia is a discrete seizure type has been unequivocally documented with video-EEG recordings.[23,174,176-179] The symptom of perioral myoclonia may also rarely occur in absence seizures of other IGEs and, as such, perioral myoclonia alone cannot be taken as sole evidence of the syndrome of PMA. However, there is often a non-fortuitous clustering of other symptoms indicating that these absences may often constitute the main symptom of a syndrome within the broad spectrum of IGE, which we proposed to call PMA. Other manifestations of this syndrome include GTCSs, which often start early prior to or together with the absences; frequent occurrence of absence status epilepticus; resistance to treatment; and persistence in adult life.[174,175]

Demographic Data

Onset varies from 2 to 13 years (median 10 years). Girls are far more frequently affected than boys. The prevalence of PMA is small in children (<1% with typical absences) but, because it fails to remit, it is higher in adults (9.3%) with TAS.

Clinical Manifestations

TAS with perioral myoclonia are the defining symptom. The characteristic feature is perioral myoclonia, which consists of rhythmic contractions of the orbicularis oris muscle that cause protrusion of the lips, contractions of the depressor anguli oris resulting in twitching of the corners of the mouth or, rarely, more widespread involvement, including the muscles of mastication producing jaw jerking (Fig. 10.1). Impairment of consciousness varies from severe to mild. Most patients are usually aware of the perioral myoclonia. Duration is usually brief, lasting a mean of 4 s (range 2–9 s). Absences of perioral myoclonia may be very frequent, occurring many times per day, 1–2 per week, or they are rare.

All patients suffer GTCSs, which often start before or soon after the onset of clinically apparent absences. Exceptionally, GTCSs may start many years

C.P. Panayiotopoulos, *Idiopathic Generalised Epilepsies*,
DOI 10.1007/978-1-4471-4039-9_10, © Springer-Verlag London 2012

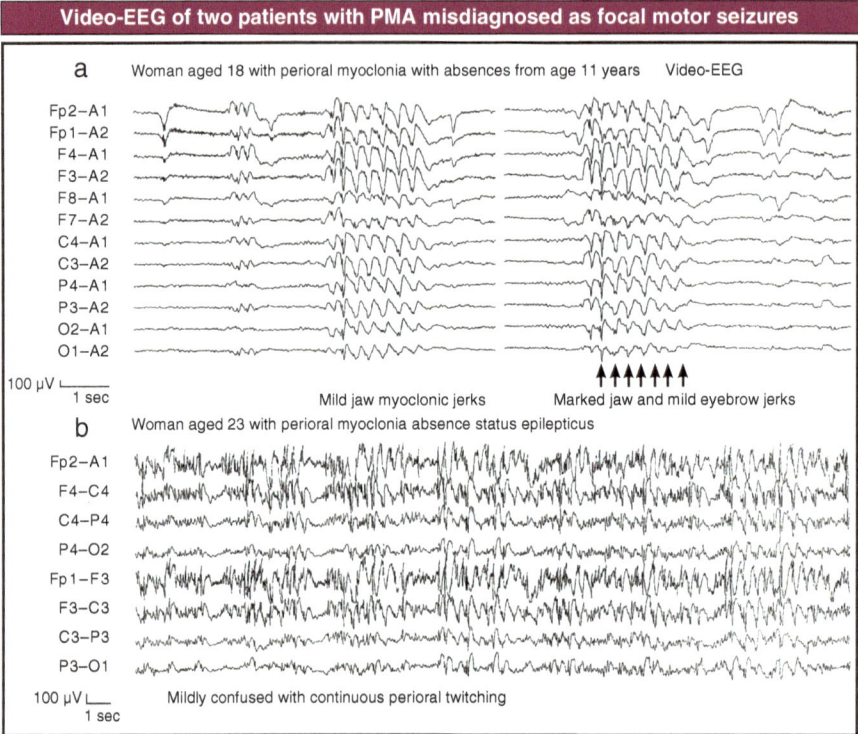

Video-EEG of two patients with PMA misdiagnosed as focal motor seizures

a   Woman aged 18 with perioral myoclonia with absences from age 11 years   Video-EEG

Mild jaw myoclonic jerks   Marked jaw and mild eyebrow jerks

b   Woman aged 23 with perioral myoclonia absence status epilepticus

Mildly confused with continuous perioral twitching

Fig. 10.1 (**a**) From video-EEG recording of a woman with perioral myoclonia with absences (case 6 in Panayiotopoulos et al.[174]). She was referred because of 'focal motor seizures and secondarily GTCS'. She had onset of GTCSs and absences at age 11 years. Seizures continued despite treatment with appropriate AED combinations such as valproate, ethosuximide, clonazepam, lamotrigine and acetazolamide. Absences were frequent, often in daily clusters and consisted of brief, about 5 s, moderate impairment of consciousness with violent rhythmic jerking of the jaw. GTCSs occurred between one and ten times per year, usually after awakening, preceded by clusters of absences with the jaw myoclonus spreading to limb jerks prior to generalised convulsions. She was more concerned about the absences because they interfered with her daily life 'everyone notices the jerks of my jaw' and less with the GTCSs, which usually occurred at home. The initial misdiagnosis of 'focal motor seizures' was because the jaw jerking was described by her mother as unilateral. (**b**) From the EEG of a 23-year-old woman while in perioral myoclonia absence status epilepticus (case 2 in Panayiotopoulos[174]). She was mildly confused with continuous perioral twitching. This ended with a GTCS. Initial presentation at age 11 years was with GTCS. Absences with perioral myoclonia were noted at the same time and were diagnosed as focal motor seizures

after the onset of absences. GTCSs are usually infrequent (range once per lifetime to 12 per year) and are often heralded by clusters of absences or absence status epilepticus.

Absence status epilepticus is very common in PMA (57%) and frequently ends with a GTCS (Fig. 10.1). It is more common than in any other syndromes of IGE with typical absences.[94] Perioral myoclonia may be more apparent than impairment of consciousness or *vice versa*.

Aetiology

Half of patients have first-degree relatives (mainly siblings) with IGE and absences.[174,180]

Diagnostic Procedures

All tests are normal except EEG.

Electroencephalography

Inter-ictal EEG frequently shows (1) abortive bursts or brief <1 s of 4–7 Hz GPSWD – these are usually asymmetrical and may give the impression of a localised focus and (2) focal abnormalities, including single spikes, spike–wave complexes and theta waves with variable side emphasis.

The ictal EEG consists of 3–4 Hz GPSWD with frequent intradischarge irregularities in terms of numbers of spike in the spike–wave complex, fluctuations in spike amplitude and the occurrence of fragmentations.

There is no photosensitivity.

Diagnostic Tips

- Useful clinical indicators in favour of PMA and against CAE, JAE or other forms of IGE:
- Onset of GTCSs before or at the same age as typical absences
- Relatively brief duration of absences with perioral myoclonia
- Frequent occurrence of absence status epilepticus

Differential Diagnosis

Patients with PMA are frequently erroneously diagnosed as having focal motor seizures, because of (1) the prominent motor features of the absences which are often reported and sometimes recorded as unilateral and (2) inter-ictal focal EEG abnormalities. However, this error is unlikely to happen if the EEG is properly obtained and interpreted. Also, patients with focal motor seizures are unlikely to suffer status epilepticus, which is common in PMA.

The main differential diagnosis is from CAE, JAE or IGE with phantom absences depending on the age at onset. Video-EEG invariably reveals perioral myoclonia that sometimes may be subtle, particularly in treated patients.

Prognosis

Absences and GTCSs may be resistant to medication, unremitting and possibly lifelong.

Management

Treatment is with valproate alone or combined with ethosuximide, small doses of lamotrigine or clonazepam.

Absence status epilepticus, for which most patients are aware, should be terminated with immediate self-administered medication of oral midazolam or rectal benzodiazepines.

IGE with Phantom Absences[159]

Phantom absences are typical absence seizures with the mildest form of impairment of consciousness.[159]

IGE with phantom absences[159,160] is characterised by a triad of:

1. Phantom absences
2. GTCSs, which are commonly the first overt clinical manifestations, usually starting in adulthood and are infrequent
3. Absence status epilepticus, which occurs in half of the patients.

Considerations on Classification

Phantom absences are mild absence seizures, causing only inconspicuous impairment of cognition. Although not classical, they fulfil the ILAE criteria of TAS with GPSWD of more than 2.5 Hz.[55,159]

Phantom absences have not been considered in any previous ILEA classification,[21,25] but this may now change. The recent ILAE report[26] makes the following reference: "Phantom absences are likely to be a result of brain maturation".

Furthermore, there is reasonable evidence to support that phantom absences are not only a discrete seizure but may also constitute the main symptom of a syndrome within the broad spectrum of IGE. There is non-fortuitous clustering of other symptoms such as GTCSs of usually late onset, frequent occurrence of absence status epilepticus and persistence into adult life.[159] That these patients have IGE is beyond any doubt as they all are of normal intelligence and physical state, high-resolution MRI is normal, the EEG shows GPSWD and the seizures are generalised.

The syndrome of IGE with phantom absences has not been recognised by the ILAE.[21,25] Accordingly, these cases are probably categorised among undefined IGE or other syndromes of IGE.

Demographic Data

The first overt clinical manifestations of GTCSs appear in adult life, although absences may have started much earlier. Men and women are equally affected. Prevalence has been estimated at 15% among IGE with typical absences, 10% of IGE and 3% of 410 consecutive patients older than 16 years with epileptic

C.P. Panayiotopoulos, *Idiopathic Generalised Epilepsies*,
DOI 10.1007/978-1-4471-4039-9_11, © Springer-Verlag London 2012

seizures.[159] Genton[181] reported that, among 253 consecutive cases of IGE, 32 (15.4%) patients had rare GTCSs with GPSWD in the inter-ictal EEG.

Clinical Manifestations

This syndrome manifests with phantom absences, GTCSs and, often, ASE.

Phantom absences denote TAS, which are so mild that they are inconspicuous to the patient and imperceptible to the observer.[159] They are disclosed by video-EEG recording and breath counting during hyperventilation. The absences manifest with interruption, delays or errors of counting and occasionally with eyelid blinking. Ictal EEG shows brief (usually 3 or 4 s), 3–4 Hz GPSWD (Fig. 11.1 and 11.2). Phantom absences may be more common than appreciated in patients with IGE (particularly adults) but are often unrecognised.

GTCSs are usually the first overt clinical manifestation.[159] These are of late onset, infrequent and without consistent circadian distribution or specific precipitating factors.

Absence status epilepticus: Half of patients suffer from absence status epilepticus, which often lasts for many hours alone or prior to a GTCS (Fig. 11.1). This manifests with cognitive impairment, which is usually of mild or moderate severity. The patient communicates poorly, is slow, feels strange and confused, makes errors at work, looks depressed but does not become unresponsive. More commonly than usually appreciated are experiential, mental and sensational symptoms. The patient is often aware of the impeding GTCS and tries to find a safe place to have it. There may be some post-ictal recollection of the events.

Aetiology

IGE with phantom absences is probably genetically determined.[159]

Diagnostic Procedures

All tests are normal except the EEG.

Electroencephalography

The background activity is normal but half of patients have EEG focal paroxysmal abnormalities consisting of short transient localised slow, sharp waves or spikes or both, occurring either independently or in association with the generalised discharges.[159,182] EEG photosensitivity is exceptional.

Ictal EEG consists of 3–4 Hz GPSWD with occasional fragmentations (Fig. 11.1 and 11.2). They are typically brief (2–4 s) lasting usually no more than 5 s. Mild cognitive impairment manifested by hesitation, discontinuation and errors in breath counting is the only clinical ictal symptom during the generalised discharges. A few patients may also have mild ictal eyelid fluttering.[159,182] Hyperventilation is a major provocative factor.

From video-EEG of IGE with phantom absences, absence status epilepticus and GTCSs

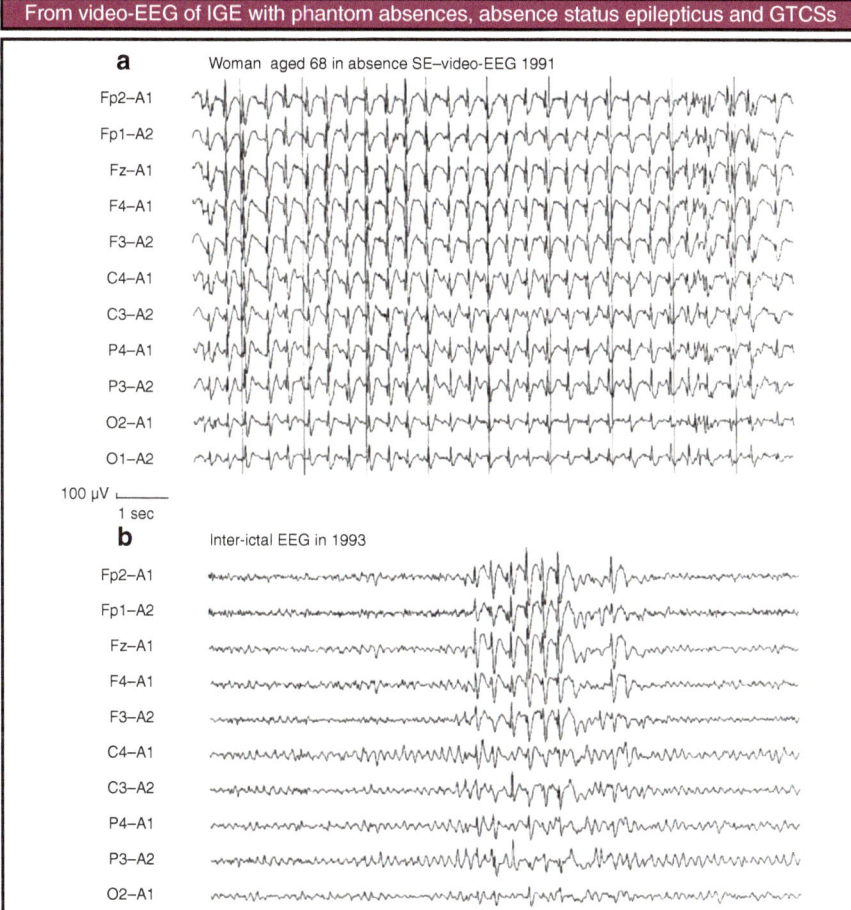

a   Woman aged 68 in absence SE–video-EEG 1991

b   Inter-ictal EEG in 1993

Fig. 11.1 From video-EEG of a highly intelligent woman, aged 76 years, with phantom absences, absence SE and GTCSs. She had her first overt seizure at age 30 years. She was moderately confused for 12 h prior to a GTCS. Since then she had between one and three similar episodes every year. She was misdiagnosed with temporal lobe epilepsy and was on primidone and sulthiame for nearly 40 years. Retrospectively, she admits to brief episodes of mild impairment of cognition. 'The absences lasted a couple of seconds; the other state [absence status] was much longer, for 24 h or more… They may be linked I suppose'. No further seizures of any type occurred in the next 11 years of follow-up on monotherapy with valproate 1,000 mg daily. (**a**) Absence SE. There was continuous slow GSWD mainly at 3 Hz. Note also slower or faster components and some topographic variability of the discharge. The patient was fully alert, attentive and cooperative. Movements and speech were normal. There were no abnormal ictal symptoms other than severe global memory deficit and global diminution of content of consciousness. She was unable to remember her name, how many children she had, date and location. She could not perform simple calculations but could repeat up to five numbers given to her. She could read text correctly and she rightly wrote her address, although she could not remember it on verbal questioning. She did not know where she was but, given the choice between various locations, she correctly recognised that she was in the hospital. This absence SE was successfully terminated with intravenous administration of diazepam. (**b**) Inter-ictal video-EEG showing brief 3 Hz GPSWD lasting 2 or 3 s without apparent clinical manifestations

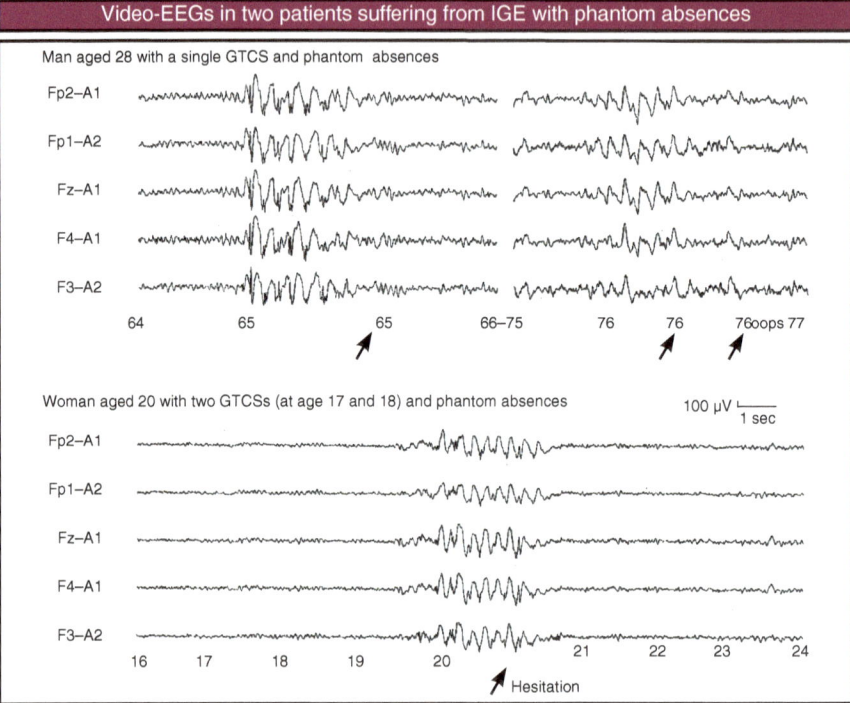

Fig. 11.2 The numbers denote the actual breath counting during hyperventilation. Note that errors, when they occur (*arrows*), are only related to these brief discharges. Errors consist of hesitation in pronouncing the next consecutive number, repetitions and erroneous counting sequence. These absences are impossible to detect without breath counting and video-EEG

During absence status epilepticus, the EEG shows continuous 3 Hz GPSWD (particularly adults) (Fig. 11.1).

Differential Diagnosis

The diagnostic and management errors involved in adult patients with IGE and TAS have been well reported.[102,159] The magnitude of the problem is worse in IGE with phantom absences, in which the absences are very mild, absence status epilepticus is misdiagnosed as non-epileptic events or temporal lobe epilepsy, and GTCSs are of late onset. This is compounded by frequent EEG focal abnormalities and the current practice of most EEG departments not to appropriately test cognition during brief GPSWD.[55]

The main features to consider in IGE with phantom absences are:

- The first overt unprovoked GTCS appears in adult life
- Absence status epilepticus
- Differentiation from other syndromes of IGE

It is essential to take a careful clinical history and to interpret symptoms correctly, which may be suggestive of typical absences and absence status epilepticus.

A history of altered consciousness preceding GTCSs should not be taken as evidence of complex focal seizures, depression or an unspecified seizure prodrome. Absence status epilepticus is more likely.

Other forms of the so-called 'adult-onset IGE' may be otherwise typical examples of JME, JAE or other IGE syndromes that start or become clinically identifiable after the age of 20 years.[183,184] Some of the patients described may suffer from IGE with phantom absences.

IGE with phantom absences is also different from IGE with GTCS. In IGE with GTCS, phantom absences do not occur, GTCSs tend to occur on awakening and episodes of absence status affect half as many patients than of IGE with phantom absences. There is no evidence for a maturational influence on the duration of GSW in either syndrome.[160]

Prognosis

IGE with phantom absences may be a lifelong propensity to seizures that is of undetermined onset and remission. Patients are of normal intelligence, which does not show any signs of deterioration. In addition, phantom absences, although frequent, do not appear to affect daily activity.

Management

There are many questions to answer in deciding whether patients with phantom absences need treatment. All patients of IGE with phantom absences had a normal life without medication until their first GTCS, probably many years after the onset of frequent daily mild absence seizures. We do not know how many people in the general population with the same problem will never develop GTCSs or absence status epilepticus. However, for those that will eventually have GTCSs, treatment may be needed. Drugs of choice are those of IGE with absence seizures; these include valproate and lamotrigine.

Absence status epilepticus should be terminated with self-administered buccal midazolam.

Autosomal Dominant Cortical Tremor, Myoclonus and Epilepsy

IGE syndromes with Mendelian (monogenic) inheritance have been described in the past decade. Of those with autosomal dominant inheritance, 'autosomal dominant cortical tremor, myoclonus and epilepsy' (ADCME) is the more common.[185-188] Familial infantile myoclonic epilepsy is of autosomal recessive inheritance.[189,190]

ADCME is a term used recently to include a number of familial autosomal disorders manifesting with cortical tremor, myoclonus and epilepsy, such as benign familial adult myoclonic epilepsy, familial adult myoclonic epilepsy, familial essential myoclonus and epilepsy, familial cortical tremor and epilepsy, and autosomal dominant cortical myoclonus and epilepsy. It has been described mainly in Japanese and Italian families. They all have a similar phenotype and the condition may be a single relatively benign non-progressive autosomal dominant IGE syndrome with high penetrance and genetic heterogeneity.[185,186,191] Its categorisation by some authors[192] among progressive myoclonus epilepsy is questionable.

Epidemiology

Age at onset of cortical tremor and myoclonus varies from 11 to 50 years. ADCME is probably the most common of all autosomal IGE syndromes.

Aetiology

ADCME, as the name suggests, is of autosomal dominant inheritance with high penetrance and genetic heterogeneity. The genes for ADCME have been mapped to 8q24 in Japanese[193,194] and 2p11.1-q12.2 in European families.[185,186,195] Conversely, none of these loci were found in a large French family with ADCME linked to chromosome 16pl3.[188]

Clinical Manifestations

Adult-onset cortical tremor and myoclonus are the defining symptoms. Cortical tremor looks like fine shivering of the fingers and hands intensified by posture, fine movement, and emotional and physical stress. The majority of patients also suffer from cortical myoclonus manifesting with distal, arrhythmic and erratic jerks of mainly the hands and fingers. These are also

C.P. Panayiotopoulos, *Idiopathic Generalised Epilepsies*,
DOI 10.1007/978-1-4471-4039-9_12, © Springer-Verlag London 2012

exaggerated by posture, fine movement, and emotional and physical stress. Most patients (80%) also have infrequent GTCSs in periods of worsening myoclonus. GTCSs are usually precipitated by sleep deprivation and photic stimulation. Rarely, in some families, additional complex focal seizures may occur. Mental and neurological states are usually normal. Families with members having concurrent migraine or blindness have been reported.

Diagnostic Procedures

The EEG shows generalised polyspikes and waves and photoparoxysmal responses. Photomyogenic responses may also be present. Somatosensory and visually evoked potentials are of very high amplitude. Consistent with cortical myoclonus, long-loop C-reflexes are enhanced and cortical spikes precede the rhythmic jerk on jerk–locked EEG back-averaging.[186] Surface EMG shows irregular, arrhythmic or semirhythmic EMG bursts at around 10 Hz. These EMG bursts last about 50 ms and are usually synchronous between agonist and antagonist muscles, without the regular agonist/antagonist alternation of the essential tremor.[185,186]

Prognosis

ADCME is a non-progressive disorder. Epileptic seizures are usually infrequent, but cortical tremor and myoclonus may sometimes be severe. Occasionally, mental decline is reported in old age.

Differential Diagnosis

Cortical tremor may be misinterpreted as essential tremor from which it is clinically and electrophysiologically different.

Management

This is with AEDs that have anti-myoclonic activity, such as valproate, phenobarbital, clonazepam and levetiracetam.[7,185,186,196] Piracetam in high doses is often beneficial for the cortical tremor. Lamotrigine, gabapentin, tiagabine and pregabalin, because of promyoclonic action, are contraindicated.

Genetic counselling, as with the autosomal dominant disorders, is part of the management.

AED Treatment of IGEs[11,12,17,23]

IGEs demand different treatment strategies from the focal epilepsies.[11,12,17,23] Ignoring this fact results in avoidable intractability, morbidity and sometimes mortality. Nearly half of patients with IGEs are treated with inappropriate AEDs. Practising physicians have a colossal task in not only properly diagnosing IGE, but also in deciding which of the many older and newer AEDs are the most suitable (Tables 13.1 and 13.2) and which are contraindicated (Table 13.3) for the seizures and preferably the syndromes of IGEs.

Seizures/syndromes	First-line AEDs[a] (in order of priority)	Second-line AEDs[a] (in order of priority)
Focal (simple and complex) seizures with or without secondarily GTCSs	Carbamazepine, phenytoin, phenobarbital	Clobazam, valproate
	Levetiracetam, oxcarbazepine, lamotrigine, topiramate	*Lacosamide, gabapentin, zonisamide, pregabalin, tiagabine*
Primarily GTCSs only	Valproate, phenobarbital, phenytoin	Carbamazepine
	Levetiracetam, lamotrigine, topiramate	*Oxcarbazepine*
Myoclonic seizures only	Clonazepam, valproate, phenobarbital	Phenytoin, ethosuximide
	Levetiracetam	*Topiramate, zonisamide*
Absence seizures only (typical and atypical)	Valproate, ethosuximide	Clonazepam
	Lamotrigine	*Levetiracetam, zonisamide, topiramate*
Negative myoclonic and atonic seizures	Ethosuxide, valproate	Clonazepam
	Levetiracetam	*Zonisamide, topiramate*
Tonic seizures	Valproate, phenytoin, phenobarbital	Clonazepam, clobazam
	Topiramate, lamotrigine	*Zonisamide*
Benign childhood focal seizures and syndromes	Carbamazepine, valproate, sulthiame, clobazam	
	Levetiracetam, oxcarbazepine, lamotrigine	*Gabapentin, lacosamide, zonisamide*

Table 13.1 Pragmatic recommendations for AED treatment with older (*black font*) and newer (*blue font*) AEDs for epileptic seizures and main epileptic syndromes

C.P. Panayiotopoulos, *Idiopathic Generalised Epilepsies*, DOI 10.1007/978-1-4471-4039-9_13, © Springer-Verlag London 2012

Seizures/syndromes	First-line AEDs[a] (in order of priority)	Second-line AEDs[a] (in order of priority)
All symptomatic and cryptogenic syndromes of focal epilepsies	Carbamazepine, phenytoin, phenobarbital	Clobazam, valproate
	Levetiracetam, oxcarbazepine, lamotrigine, topiramate	*Lacosamide, gabapentin, zonisamide, pregabalin, tiagabine*
Childhood absence epilepsy	Ethosuxide, valproate	Clonazepam
	Lamotrigine	
Juvenile absence epilepsy	Valproate, ethosuximide	Clonazepam
	Lamotrigine	*Levetiracetam, zonisamide, topiramate*
Juvenile myoclonic epilepsy	Valproate, phenobarbital	Clonazepam, ethosuximide
	Levetiracetam, topiramate	*Zonisamide, lamotrigine*
Photosensitive and other reflex seizures	Valproate	Clonazepam
	Levetiracetam	*Lamotrigine*
Lennox–Gastaut syndrome and other epileptic encephalopathies (AEDs largely depend on predominant seizure type)	Valproate	Clobazam, clonazepam, ethosuximide, phenytoin
	Lamotrigine, levetiracetam, rufinamide, topiramide, zonisamide	*Felbamate, stiripentol (Dravet syndrome only)*

[a]Older AEDs are shown in roman black font; newer AEDs are shown in blue italics. The table is only indicative of AEDs to use in each of the epileptic seizures or syndromes. Priority depends on AED properties, whether monotherapy or polytherapy is used, and the needs of individual patients, as detailed in this book. In choosing an AED from this table, the order of priority is between the first in the list of older or newer AEDs in the middle column

Table 13.1 (continued)

The management of women with IGEs at childbearing age has been significantly affected by the revelations of valproate adverse reactions and its practical exclusion in this specified group of patients. What are the alternatives?

Important clinical facts to remember are:

- GTCSs are the more likely cause of referral. The first task of the physician is to properly diagnose whether these are of generalised onset (primarily GTCSs) or of focal-onset (secondarily GTCSs), which have different responses to AED treatment. Table 13.4 lists AEDs licensed for the prophylactic treatment of primarily GTCSs in the USA or Europe or both. AEDs licensed and recommended for secondarily GTCSs are listed in Chapter 15.
- Absences and myoclonic jerks are other types of seizure in IGEs that should be detected. These may often occur long before the first GTCS and/or may be the main seizures, as for example with absences of CAE and JAE, and the myoclonic jerks of JME.
- Photosensitivity is a common precipitating or facilitating factor of seizures occurring in a third of patients with IGEs.

AED	Myoclonic jerks	GTCSs	Absences	Photo-sensitivity	Serious ADRs[a]	Titration	Drug–drug interactions[b]
Valproate	Very effective	Very effective	Very effective	Very effective	Yes	Optional (2–4 weeks)	Many
Levetiracetam	Very effective	Very effective	Effective	Very effective	No	Optional (1–2 weeks)[c]	Insignificant[d]
Lamotrigine	Exaggerates in 50 %	Very effective	Very effective	Probablyeffective	Yes	Mandatory (6–8 weeks)	Many
Topiramate	Probably effective	Very effective	Probably effective	Undetermined	Yes	Mandatory (6–8 weeks	Many
Clonazepam	Very effective	Ineffective	Weakly effective	Weaklyeffective	No	Mandatory (3–4 weeks)	Insignificant
Ethosuximide	Effective (negative myoclonus)	Ineffective	Very effective	Ineffective	Yes	Mandatory(3–4 weeks)	Insignificant
Zonisamide	Effective	Effective	Weakly effective	Ineffective	Yes	Mandatory (4–5 weeks)	Many
Phenobarbital	Effective	Very effective	Ineffective	Ineffective	Yes	Mandatory (6–8 weeks)	Many

[a]See references 196a, 197, 198

[b]See references 196a, 199

[c]Sometimes the first dose is therapeutic

[d]Enzyme inducers may decrease its plasma levels by 20–30

Table 13.2 Efficacy and safety of primary AEDs used in the treatment of IGEs, the triad of their seizures and photosensitivity

Carbamazepine, oxcarbazepine and phenytoin (though they may control primarily GTCS if added to first-line drugs)
Gabapentin (ineffective in primarily GTCS and may exacerbate absences and myoclonic jerks)
Pregabalin (strongly pro-myoclonic)
Tiagabine and vigabatrin (strongly pro-absence drugs with a high incidence of induced absence status epilepticus)

[a]Contraindicated is any AED that either makes seizures worse or is ineffective because (1) it averts beneficial AED treatment or (2) it exposes the patient to unnecessary ADRs (some of which may be life threatening) with no benefit to the illness

Table 13.3 AED contraindicated in the treatment of IGEs[a]

AEDs licensed for primarily GTCSs (sole or adjunctive)	Other types of seizure
Carbamazepine	Exaggerates absences and myoclonic jerks
Clonazepam	Also licensed for absences and myoclonic jerks but may exaggerate GTCSs in JME
Lamotrigine	Also licensed for absences but exaggerates myoclonic jerks
Levetiracetam	Also licensed for myoclonic jerks
Phenobarbital	Also licensed for myoclonic jerks but exaggerates absences
Phenytoin	Exaggerates absences and myoclonic jerks
Primidone	Also licensed for myoclonic jerks but exaggerates absences
Topiramate	Not licensed for absences or myoclonic jerks
Valproate	Also licensed for absences and myoclonic jerks

Table 13.4 AEDs licensed (FDA, EMEA or both) for the prophylactic treatment of primarily GTCSs

Important established documentation to remember is that:
(A) Many AEDs licensed for the treatment of focal epilepsies are contraindicated in IGEs (Table 13.3).
- Tiagabine and vigabatrin are major pro-absence agents
- Carbamazepine, oxcarbazepine and phenytoin exacerbate absences and myoclonic jerks
- Gabapentin and pregabalin are ineffective in all types of idiopathic epileptic seizures and may exacerbate some of them, particularly myoclonic jerks.
(B) A drug efficacious in one type of generalised seizure may be ineffective or exaggerate another type of generalised seizure. Even among the AEDs licensed for the treatment of primarily GTCSs (Table 13.4):
- Carbamazepine, oxcarbazepine and phenytoin exacerbate absences and myoclonic jerks

- Clonazepam is the best choice of drug for myoclonic jerks, but is ineffective in primarily GTCSs
- Lamotrigine is effective in primarily GTCSs and absences, but may exacerbate myoclonic jerks.[150,151,200,201]

(C) A drug efficacious in 'generalised' seizures of childhood epileptic encephalopathies may be ineffective or exaggerate IGEs:
- Vigabatrin is the drug of first choice in the treatment of West syndrome, but its use is contraindicated in IGE.

(D) A drug found to be efficacious in secondarily GTCSs may be ineffective in primarily GTCSs or deleterious in IGEs:
- Gabapentin and pregabalin are AEDs licensed for 'the treatment of focal and secondarily GTCSs', are ineffective in primarily GTCSs and may aggravate other types of IGE seizures, particularly myoclonic jerks
- Tiagabine, an AED licensed for the treatment of focal and secondarily GTCSs, is a potent pro-absence agent that induces absence seizures and provokes absence status epilepticus, often ending with GTCSs in IGE.

(E) In patients with primarily GTCSs, an AED that abolishes another type of seizure (i.e. absences or myoclonic jerks) does not necessarily reduce the frequency of primarily GTCSs. This contrasts with secondarily GTCSs, where AEDs that abolish focal seizures also eradicate secondarily GTCSs:
- Ethosuximide is a first option AED for absence seizures and negative myoclonus but is ineffective in GTCSs
- Clonazepam is the most effective anti-myoclonic AED, but its effect in absences is weak and may aggravate GTCSs.

(F) IGEs are often easily treatable, which means that a small dose of an appropriate AED is as good as a large dose.[202]
- No difference in the control of various types of JME could be demonstrated between 1,000 mg and 2,000 mg of valproate.[203]

Treatment of Newly Diagnosed IGEs

The treatment of newly diagnosed patients with IGEs should follow the same general principles detailed in Chapter 7 of reference 196a. Diagnosis should first establish that the patient has genuine epileptic seizures and then:
- Ensure that this is IGE and not focal epilepsy
- Define the types of seizure that the patient suffers in order of severity and risk to the patient
- Define, if possible, the IGE syndrome

In choosing the first AED to be recommended from Table 13.2, efficacy and adverse reactions have to be carefully balanced, because treatment is often lifelong. Therefore, also consider long-term effects such as:
- Adverse drug reactions (ADRs) on growth and development of children
- Hormonal changes and ADRs on the reproductive life of a woman, including teratogenicity

The management and AED treatment specific to each syndrome of IGE can be found in the description of the epileptic syndromes of this chapter.

IGEs: RCTs and Evidence-Based Recommendations

There is an especially alarming lack of well-designed, properly conducted RCTs for patients with generalised seizures/epilepsies and for children in general.[205]

In the 2006 ILAE authoritative evidence-based review and analysis of the efficacy and effectiveness of AEDs as initial monotherapy for epileptic seizures,[205] no AED reached the high level A (AED established as efficacious or effective) or B (probably efficacious or effective) required for an AED to 'be considered for initial monotherapy – first-line monotherapy' in:

- Adults and children with GTCSs
- Children with absence seizures
- Juvenile myoclonic epilepsy.

Myoclonic seizures or other IGEs could not even be assessed.

Clinical Note

Do all primarily GTCSs of different syndromes have the same responsiveness?[12]

It is postulated, but not proven, that primarily GTCSs of idiopathic epilepsies are all equally responsive to the various AEDs.[12] This is probable for primarily GTCSs of IGEs. However, primarily GTCSs of febrile seizures are mainly responsive to phenobarbital and valproate, but not to carbamazepine and phenytoin.

It is likely, but not proven, that primarily GTCSs of symptomatic epilepsies do not have the same responsiveness as the primarily GTCSs of IGEs. Knowing the answer to these questions may have a significant impact in the interpretation of certain RCTs and particularly those that have studied the effect of an AED in so-called primarily GTCSs in mixed populations of IGEs and symptomatic generalised epilepsies; e.g. in an RCT evaluating topiramate for primarily GTCS, almost half (41 %) of patients had tonic seizures (24 %), atypical absences (8 %) and drop attacks (9 %), none of which are types of seizure accepted in IGEs.204 Furthermore, to emphasise the diagnostic problems in these studies, one patient included in the topiramate analysis group was diagnosed as having Lennox–Gastaut syndrome based on information obtained after study completion.[204]

In a recent class 3 RCT involving patients with IGE,[206] valproate was significantly better than both lamotrigine (hazard ratio [HR] 1.55; 95% confidence interval [CI], 1.07–2.24) and topiramate (HR 1.89; 95% CI, 1.32–2.70) for time to treatment failure. For time to 12-month remission, valproate was significantly better than lamotrigine (HR 0.68; 95% CI, 0.53–0.89), but there was no significant difference between valproate and topiramate. Levetiracetam has not been assessed.

In addition to other methodological problems, this RCT did not study the effects of the AEDs on the different seizure types of IGE (absences, myoclonic jerks or GTCSs) or IGE syndromes. This contradicts the aforementioned principles of AED therapy of IGEs, which are in agreement with the authors' statement: 'an overall analysis, ignoring epilepsy type, might lead to an erroneous conclusion that a new drug is not inferior to a standard'.[206] In addition, like in all other RCTs, 'misclassification of patients' epilepsy type'[207] and 'questionable selection of patients'[208] may have confounded the results of RCTs examining the effect of AEDs in IGE, particularly on primarily GTCSs.

For the levels of evidence supporting the recommendations proposed in this section, see Chapter 7 of reference 196a.

Older AEDs in IGEs[11,23]

Of the older AEDs effective in the treatment of IGEs the position is as follows (the AEDs are listed in order of efficacy in primarily GTCSs).

Valproate has superior efficacy in all seizures and syndromes of IGEs. Valproate monotherapy controls absence seizures and myoclonic jerks in about 75% and GTCSs in 70 % of patients with IGE. Valproate is the first-choice AED in IGEs for men. However, valproate is undesirable in women because of its teratogenic effects and its tendency to cause weight gain and polycystic ovary syndrome (see Principles of therapy in women with epilepsy; Chapter 7 of reference 196a). The risk for major congenital malformations (MCMs) with valproate monotherapy is three to five times higher than the background rate. This is higher with increasing doses of valproate, and it is double or more in combination with other AEDs, particularly with lamotrigine (10%).[209,210]

Phenobarbital is the preferred drug for the treatment of primarily GTCSs and JME when cost is of concern. It worsens absences.

Phenytoin is effective in primarily GTCSs. It worsens absences and possibly myoclonic jerks.

Carbamazepine is effective in primarily GTCSs, but aggravates absences and myoclonic jerks.

Clonazepam, even in small doses of 0.5–1 mg, is probably the most potent antimyoclonic drug with some anti-absence effect; it is ineffective in primarily GTCSs or, by suppressing myoclonic jerks, deprive patients of the warning symptoms of an impeding GTCS.[157]

Clobazam has not been evaluated in primarily GTCSs of IGE, but it may be effective in some cases. Clobazam is a very useful AED in focal epilepsies and secondarily GTCSs. However, in IGE, I have found clobazam to be far inferior to clonazepam in controlling myoclonic jerks, and may have only a very weak effect on absences.

Acetazolamide has been used for treating primarily GTCSs in cases resistant to conventional treatment, although its use may induce nephrolithiasis.[211]

Ethosuximide is a potent anti-absence AED controlling 70% of absences in monotherapy. It may improve myoclonic seizures (particularly negative epileptic myoclonus), but is ineffective in GTCSs.

Newer AEDs Useful in IGEs

Of the newer AEDs, only levetiracetam, lamotrigine, topiramate and zonisamide (in order of efficacy) appear to be effective agents in IGEs. All others – vigabatrin, tiagabine, gabapentin, pregabalin and oxcarbazepine – are contraindicated in IGEs.

Levetiracetam, because of its efficacy in primarily GTCSs,[103] myoclonic jerks[104] and photosensitivity and its safer ADR profile, appears to be the most probable substitute for valproate in at least JME and women.[146–148,212,213]

Of significant importance in the treatment of women with IGEs are the reported results of the UK Pregnancy Registry (see Table 13.5).[214]

Lamotrigine is effective in primarily GTCSs[215] and absence seizures,[205] whereas it aggravates myoclonic jerks.[151] It has important pharmacodynamic interactions with valproate. Problems with lamotrigine include a high incidence of idiosyncratic reactions that are more prominent in children and can occasionally be fatal; marked interactions with pregnancy[153,155,216] and

	Number of women with epilepsy	MCM (%)	95% CI
No exposure to AEDs	445	2.2	1.2–4.1
Exposure to AEDs	5475	3.9	3.4–7.2
Monotherapy	4276	3.4	2.9–4.9
Polytherapy (> 130 AED combinations)	1199	5.8	4.6–7.2
Polytherapy with valproate[a]	451	8.6	6.4–11.6
Polytherapy with carbamazepine	526	4.9	3.4–7.1
Polytherapy with lamotrigine	644	5.3	3.8–7.3
Polytherapy with levetiracetam	229	3.9	2.1–7.3
Polytherapy with topiramate	162	8.6	5.2–14.0
Monotherapy with valproate	1097	5.8	4.5–7.4
Monotherapy with carbamazepine	1444	2.4	1.7–3.3
Monotherapy with lamotrigne	1524	2.4	1.7–3.3
Monotherapy with levetiracetam	177	0	0.0–2.3
Monotherapy with topiramate	92	4.8	1.9–7.6

Data courtesy of Dr Jim Morrow and the UK Epilepsy and Pregnancy Register. For recent monotherapy data from the North American AED register (which do not differ significantly from those of the UK) please see http://www2.mass-general.org/aed/newsletter/Winter2009newsletter.pdf.
[a]Polytherapy with valproate had a significantly higher rate of MCM (8.6%) than regimens without valproate (odds ratio 2.3; 95% CI 1.4–3.7). Monotherapy data updated to November 2009; all others are up to July 2009

Table 13.5 MCM in the UK Epilepsy and Pregnancy Register

hormonal contraception;[217] and possible teratogenicity (see Principles of therapy in women with epilepsy, Chapter 7 of reference 196a).[156,210]

Topiramate[218] is another broad-spectrum AED that is effective in primarily GTCSs[205] and myoclonic jerks, with some weak action on absence seizures.[219] In the IGEs, including JME, it appears to be less effective than valproate but more effective than lamotrigine.[206] Topiramate is unlikely to achieve monotherapy status in the long-term treatment of IGEs, mainly because of its many ADRs and its relatively inferior efficacy in IGEs compared with valproate and levetiracetam. More recently, concerns have also been raised about possible teratogenic effects in women with epilepsy and that in animal experiments topiramate may damage the retina, similar to vigabatrin.[220]

Zonisamide is also a broad-spectrum AED, but its role in IGE is largely uncertain.[221] It probably has a weak beneficial effect in primarily GTCSs, absences and jerks, although a few patients may have an excellent response.[222] ADRs may be particularly troublesome in children.

Monotherapy with one of the AEDs listed in Table 13.2 is unlikely to fail if it is appropriately evaluated and chosen for the particular IGE syndrome and individual patient. Monotherapy should not be abandoned before making sure that the maximum tolerated dose has been achieved.

Management of Patients with Difficult to Treat IGEs

IGEs have a better prognosis, and a more favourable response to, appropriate AEDs than symptomatic and focal epilepsies: 'most patients with IGE are easily controlled with appropriate medication, refractory patients are rare'.[223] Prevalence of intractable IGE may be in the order of 10–30% and this is mostly due to delayed or inappropriate treatment.[224]

Management of patients with difficult to treat IGEs, providing that they truly suffer from epileptic seizures, should follow the same principles as detailed in Chapter 7 of reference 196a:

- Based on clinical and EEG evidence, establish the type or types of seizures (absences, myoclonic jerks and GTCSs alone or in combination) and make sure that these are primarily and not secondarily generalised. Previous EEGs, particularly in untreated stages, are invaluable.
- Establish precipitating factors and circadian distribution as well as their effect regarding intractability.
- List in chronological order all AEDs previously used, and in what doses and combinations. Establish which drugs were beneficial and which made the situation worse.
- Consider thoroughly the current situation regarding (1) seizures – which are the more predominant and more disturbing – and (2) AEDs – which are definitely or possibly effective, ineffective or contraindicated with respect to seizures and adverse reactions.
- Consider thoroughly all the above, including sex, age and compliance, in making a definite plan of which AEDs with adverse effects (seizure

efficacy and patient tolerability) should be withdrawn and which of the indicated AEDs should be increased in dosage or added to the scheme.

- Of the newer AEDs, those which are likely to be effective as monotherapy are also the most likely to be suitable in polytherapy. The order of priority as determined by efficacy, safety, drug–drug interactions and other parameters are levetiracetam, lamotrigine, topiramate and zonisamide. All other newer AEDs – gabapentin, oxcarbazepine, pregabalin, tiagabine and vigabatrin – are contraindicated.

Drug Withdrawal

In CAE, treatment may be slowly withdrawn 1–3 years after controlling all absences. All other syndromes of the IGEs are probably lifelong and confront the usual textbook advice of withdrawal of medication after 2 or 3 years from the last seizure because relapses are probably unavoidable. However, if seizures are mild and infrequent, drug withdrawal may be attempted. This should be in small decrements, probably over years, warning the patient that re-appearance of even minor seizures such as absences or myoclonic jerks mandates continuation of treatment. EEG confirmation of the seizure-free state is needed during the withdrawal period.

Useful Reminder

Small doses of the added AED are sometimes very effective.

In cases with persistent myoclonic jerks, clonazepam in a single small dose (0.5–2 mg) prior to sleep may have a dramatic beneficial effect.[75]

In men on valproate, adding small doses of lamotrigine (25–50 mg) is very effective because of pharmacodynamic interactions between these drugs.

Management of Status Epilepticus in IGEs

IGEs have a high prevalence of absence status epilepticus, which often goes undetected or is misdiagnosed as a prodrome or focal non-convulsive status epilepticus (which is less common than absence status epilepticus).[225] Conversely, generalised tonic–clonic status epilepticus is less common in IGEs than other epilepsies.

The management of status epilepticus is detailed in Chapter 3 of reference 196a.

References

1. Jallon P, Latour P. Epidemiology of idiopathic generalized epilepsies. Epilepsia. 2005;46 Suppl 9:10–4.
2. Gardiner M. Genetics of idiopathic generalized epilepsies. Epilepsia. 2005;46 Suppl 9:15–20.
3. Duron RM, Medina MT, Martinez-Juarez I, Bailey JN, Perez-Gosiengfiao KT, Ramos-Ramirez R, et al. Seizures of idiopathic generalized epilepsies. Epilepsia. 2005;46 Suppl 9:34–47.
4. Covanis A. Photosensitivity in idiopathic generalized epilepsies. Epilepsia. 2005;46 Suppl 9:67–72.
5. Shorvon S, Walker M. Status epilepticus in idiopathic generalized epilepsy. Epilepsia. 2005;46 Suppl 9:73–9.
6. Nordli Jr DR. Idiopathic generalized epilepsies recognized by the International League Against Epilepsy. Epilepsia. 2005;46 Suppl 9:48–56.
7. Panayiotopoulos CP. Syndromes of idiopathic generalized epilepsies not recognized by the International League Against Epilepsy. Epilepsia. 2005;46 Suppl 9:57–66.
8. Ferrie CD. Idiopathic generalized epilepsies imitating focal epilepsies. Epilepsia. 2005;46 Suppl 9:91–5.
9. Oguni H. Symptomatic epilepsies imitating idiopathic generalized epilepsies. Epilepsia. 2005;46 Suppl 9:84–90.
10. Koutroumanidis M, Smith S. Use and abuse of EEG in the diagnosis of idiopathic generalized epilepsies. Epilepsia. 2005;46 Suppl 9:96–107.
11. Hitiris N, Brodie MJ. Evidence-based treatment of idiopathic generalized epilepsies with older antiepileptic drugs. Epilepsia. 2005;46 Suppl 9:149–53.
12. Bergey GK. Evidence-based treatment of idiopathic generalized epilepsies with new antiepileptic drugs. Epilepsia. 2005;46 Suppl 9:161–8.
13. Chaves J, Sander JW. Seizure aggravation in idiopathic generalized epilepsies. Epilepsia. 2005;46 Suppl 9:133–9.
14. Camfield C, Camfield P. Management guidelines for children with idiopathic generalized epilepsy. Epilepsia. 2005;46 Suppl 9:112–6.
15. Thomas P, Valton L, Genton P. Absence and myoclonic status epilepticus precipitated by antiepileptic drugs in idiopathic generalized epilepsy. Brain. 2006;129:1281–92.
16. Benbadis SR, Tatum WO, Gieron M. Idiopathic generalized epilepsy and choice of antiepileptic drugs. Neurology. 2003;61:1793–5.
17. Benbadis SR. Practical management issues for idiopathic generalized epilepsies. Epilepsia. 2005;46 Suppl 9:125–32.
18. Panayiotopoulos CP. Idiopathic generalised epilepsies: a review and modern approach. Epilepsia. 2005;46 Suppl 9:1–160.
19. Wolf P. Historical aspects of idiopathic generalized epilepsies. Epilepsia. 2005;46 Suppl 9:7–9.
20. Andermann F, Berkovic SF. Idiopathic generalized epilepsy with generalised and other seizures in adolescence. Epilepsia. 2001;42:317–20.
21. Commission on Classification and Terminology of the International League Against Epilepsy. Proposal for revised classification of epilepsies and epileptic syndromes. Epilepsia. 1989;30:389–99.
22. Panayiotopoulos CP, Obeid T, Waheed G. Differentiation of typical absence seizures in epileptic syndromes. A video EEG study of 224 seizures in 20 patients. Brain. 1989;112:1039–56.
23. Panayiotopoulos CP. Idiopathic generalised epilepsies. In: Panayiotopoulos CP, editor. The epilepsies: seizures, syndromes and management. Oxford: Bladon Medical Publishing; 2005. p. 271–348.
24. van Luijtelaar G, Coenen A. Genetic models of absence epilepsy: New concepts and insights. In: Schwartzkroin PA, editor. Encyclopedia of basic epilepsy research, vol. 1. Oxford: Elsevier; 2009. p. 1–8.
25. Engel Jr J. A proposed diagnostic scheme for people with epileptic seizures and with epilepsy: report of the ILAE Task Force on classification and terminology. Epilepsia. 2001;42:796–803.
26. Panayiotopoulos CP, editors. Idiopathic generalised epilepsies with myoclonic jerks. Oxford: Medicinae, 2007.
27. Doose H. Das akinetische petit mal. Arch Psychiatr Nervenkr. 1965;205:638–54.
28. Doose H, Baier WK. Epilepsy with primarily generalized monoclonic-astatic seizures: a genetically determined disease. Eur J Pediatr. 1987;146:550–4.
29. Doose H. Myoclonic-astatic epilepsy. Epilepsy Res Suppl. 1992;6:163–8.

30. Oguni H, Fukuyama Y, Tanaka T, Hayashi K, Funatsuka M, Sakauchi M, et al. Myoclonic-astatic epilepsy of early childhood – clinical and EEG analysis of myoclonic-astatic seizures, and discussions on the nosology of the syndrome. Brain Dev. 2001;23:757–64.
31. Scheffer IE, Wallace R, Mulley JC, Berkovic SF. Clinical and molecular genetics of myoclonic-astatic epilepsy and severe myoclonic epilepsy in infancy (Dravet syndrome). Brain Dev. 2001;23:732–5.
32. Oguni H, Hayashi K, Imai K, Funatsuka M, Sakauchi M, Shirakawa S, et al. Idiopathic myoclonic-astatic epilepsy of early childhood – nosology based on electrophysiologic and long-term follow-up study of patients. Adv Neurol. 2005;95:157–74.
33. Dreifuss F, Dulac O. Myoclonic-astatic epilepsy of childhood. http://www.ilae-epilepsy.org/Visitors/Centre/ctf/myoclonic_astatic_child.cfm. Last accessed on 12 Aug 2011.
34. Doose H, Gerken H, Leonhardt T. Centrencephalic monoclonic-astatic petit mal. Clinical and genetic investigation. Neuropadiatrie. 1970;2:59–78.
35. Stephani U. The natural history of myoclonic astatic epilepsy (doose syndrome) and lennox-gastaut syndrome. Epilepsia. 2006;47 Suppl 2:53–5.
36. Neubauer BA, Hahn A, Doose H, Tuxhorn I. Myoclonic-astatic epilepsy of early childhood – definition, course, nosography, and genetics. Adv Neurol. 2005;95:147–55.
37. Aicardi J, Levy Gomes A. Clinical and electroencephalographic symptomatology of the 'genuine' Lennox–Gastaut syndrome and its differentiation from other forms of epilepsy of early childhood. Epilepsy Res Suppl. 1992;6:185–93.
38. Kaminska A, Ickowicz A, Plouin P, Bru MF, Dellatolas G, Dulac O. Delineation of cryptogenic Lennox–Gastaut syndrome and myoclonic astatic epilepsy using multiple correspondence analysis. Epilepsy Res. 1999;36:15–29.
39. Mullen SA, Marini C, Suls A et al. Glucose transporter 1 deficiency as a treatable cause of myoclonic astatic epilepsy. Arch Neurol 2011;68:1152–5.
40. Bonanni P, Parmeggiani L, Guerrini R. Different neurophysiologic patterns of myoclonus characterize Lennox–Gastaut syndrome and myoclonic astatic epilepsy. Epilepsia. 2002;43:609–15.
41. Fejerman N, Caraballo R, Tenembaum SN. Atypical evolutions of benign localization-related epilepsies in children: are they predictable? Epilepsia. 2000;41:380–90.
42. Fejerman N. Atypical evolution of benign partial epilepsy in children. Rev Neurol. 1996;24:1415–20.
43. Ferrie CD, Koutroumanidis M, Rowlinson S, Sanders S, Panayiotopoulos CP. Atypical evolution of Panayiotopoulos syndrome: a case report [published with video sequences]. Epileptic Disord. 2002;4:35–42.
44. Caraballo RH, Astorino F, Cersosimo R, Soprano AM, Fejerman N. Atypical evolution in childhood epilepsy with occipital paroxysms (Panayiotopoulos type). Epileptic Disord. 2001;3:157–62.
45. Panayiotopoulos CP. Benign childhood partial seizures and related epileptic syndromes. London: John Libbey & Co. Ltd; 1999.
46. Chapman K, Holland K, Erenberg G. Seizure exacerbation associated with oxcarbazepine in idiopathic focal epilepsy of childhood. Neurology. 2003;61:1012.
47. Catania S, Cross H, De Sousa C, Boyd S. Paradoxic reaction to lamotrigine in a child with benign focal epilepsy of childhood with centrotemporal spikes. Epilepsia. 1999;40:1657–60.
48. Kikumoto K, Yoshinaga H, Oka M, Ito M, Endoh F, Akiyama T, et al. EEG and seizure exacerbation induced by carbamazepine in Panayiotopoulos syndrome. Epileptic Disord. 2006;8:53–6.
49. Jayawant S, Libretto SE. Topiramate in the treatment of monoclonic-astatic epilepsy in children: a retrospective hospital audit. J Postgrad Med. 2003;49:202–6.
50. Kilaru S, Bergqvist AG. Current treatment of myoclonic astatic epilepsy: clinical experience at the Children's Hospital of Philadelphia. Epilepsia. 2007;48:1703–7.
51. Caraballo RH, Cersosimo RO, Sakr D, Cresta A, Escobal N, Fejerman N. Ketogenic diet in patients with myoclonic-astatic epilepsy. Epileptic Disord. 2006;8:151–5.
52. Oguni H, Tanaka T, Hayashi K, Funatsuka M, Sakauchi M, Shirakawa S, et al. Treatment and long-term prognosis of monoclonic-astatic epilepsy of early childhood. Neuropediatrics. 2002;33:122–32.
53. Hirsch E, Panayiotopoulos CP. Childhood absence epilepsy and related syndromes. In: Roger J, Bureau M, Dravet C, et al., editors Epileptic syndromes in infancy, childhood and adolescence. Fourth edition, with video. Montrouge: John Libbey Eurotext; 2005. p. 315–35.
54. Loiseau P, Panayiotopoulos CP. Childhood absence epilepsy. http://www.ilae-epilepsy.org/Visitors/Centre/ctf/childhood_absence.html. Last accessed 12 Aug 2011.
55. Panayiotopoulos CP. Typical absence seizures and related epileptic syndromes: assessment of current state and directions for future research. Epilepsia. 2008;49:2131–9.
56. Engel Jr J. Report of the ILAE Classification Core Group. Epilepsia. 2006;47:1558–68.
57. Fong GC, Shah PU, Gee MN, Serratosa JM, Castroviejo IP, Khan S, et al. Childhood absence epilepsy with tonic-clonic seizures and electroencephalogram 3-4-Hz spike and multispike-slow wave complexes: linkage to chromosome 8q24. Am J Hum Genet. 1998;63:1117–29.
58. Wirrell EC. Natural history of absence epilepsy in children. Can J Neurol Sci. 2003;30:184–8.

59. Fakhoury T, Abou-Khalil B. Generalized absence seizures with 10-15 Hz fast discharges. Clin Neurophysiol. 1999;110:1029–35.
60. Sadleir LG, Farrell K, Smith S, Connolly MB, Scheffer IE. Electroclinical features of absence seizures in childhood absence epilepsy. Neurology. 2006;67:413–8.
61. Panayiotopoulos CP. Typical absence seizures. http://www.ilae-epilepsy.org/Visitors/Centre/ctf/typical_absence.html. Last accessed 12 Aug 2011.
62. Adie WJ. Pyknolepsy: a form of epilepsy occurring in children with a good prognosis. Brain. 1924; 47:96–102.
63. Crunelli V, Leresche N. Childhood absence epilepsy: genes, channels, neurons and networks. Nat Rev Neurosci. 2002;3:371–82.
64. Lennox WG, Lennox MA. Epilepsy and related disorders. Boston: Little, Brown & Co; 1960.
65. Marini C, Harkin LA, Wallace RH, Mulley JC, Scheffer IE, Berkovic SF. Childhood absence epilepsy and febrile seizures: a family with a GABA(A) receptor mutation. Brain. 2003;126:230–40.
66. Chen Y, Lu J, Pan H, Zhang Y, Wu H, Xu K, et al. Association between genetic variation of CACNA1H and childhood absence epilepsy. Ann Neurol. 2003;54:239–43.
67. Peloquin JB, Khosravani H, Barr W, Bladen C, Evans R, Mezeyova J, et al. Functional analysis of Ca3.2 T-type calcium channel mutations linked to childhood absence epilepsy. Epilepsia. 2006;47:655–8.
68. Guilhoto LM, Manreza ML, Yacubian EM. Occipital intermittent rhythmic delta activity in absence epilepsy. Arq Neuropsiquiatr. 2006;64:193–7.
69. Caraballo RH, Fontana E, Darra F, et al. Childhood absence epilepsy and electroencephalographic focal abnormalities with or without clinical manifestations. Seizure. 2008;17:617–24.
70. Callenbach PM, Bouma PA, Geerts AT, Arts WF, Stroink H, et al. Long-term outcome of childhood absence epilepsy: Dutch Study of Epilepsy in Childhood. Epilepsy Res. 2009;83:249–56.
71. Caplan R, Siddarth P, Stahl L, Lanphier E, Vona P, et al. Childhood absence epilepsy: behavioral, cognitive, and linguistic comorbidities. Epilepsia. 2008;49:1838–46.
72. Caplan R, Levitt J, Siddarth P, Wu KN, Gurbani S, et al. Frontal and temporal volumes in childhood absence epilepsy. Epilepsia. 2009;50:2466–72.
73. Nadler B, Shevell MI. Childhood absence epilepsy requiring more than one medication for seizure control. Can J Neurol Sci. 2008;35:297–300.
74. Posner E. Pharmacological treatment of childhood absence epilepsy. Expert Rev Neurother. 2006;6:855–62.
75. Panayiotopoulos CP. Treatment of typical absence seizures and related epileptic syndromes. Paediatr Drugs. 2001;3:379–403.
76. Frank LM, Enlow T, Holmes GL, Manasco P, Concannon S, Chen C, et al. Lamictal (lamotrigine) monotherapy for typical absence seizures in children. Epilepsia. 1999;40:973–9.
77. Coppola G, Licciardi F, Sciscio N, Russo F, Carotenuto M, Pascotto A. Lamotrigine as first-line drug in childhood absence epilepsy: a clinical and neurophysiological study. Brain Dev. 2004;26:26–9.
78. Tassinari CA, Lyagoubi S, Santos V, Gambarelli F, Roger J, Dravet C, et al. Study on spike and wave discharges in man. II. Clinical and electroencephalographic aspects of myoclonic absence. Rev Neurol (Paris). 1969;121:379–83.
79. Verrotti A, Greco R, Chiarelli F, Domizio S, Sabatino G, Morgese G. Epilepsy with myoclonic absences with early onset: a follow up study. J Child Neurol. 1999;14:746–9.
80. Tassinari CA, Rubboli G, Gardella E, et al. Epilepsy with myoclonic absences. In: Wallace SJ, Farrell K, editors. Epilepsy in children. London: Arnold; 2004. p. 189–94.
81. Bureau M, Tassinari CA. Myoclonic absences: the seizure and the syndrome. Adv Neurol. 2005;95:175–83.
82. Tassinari A, Rubolli R, Michellluchi R. Epilepsy with myoclonic absences. http://www.ilae-epilepsy.org/Visitors/Centre/ctf/myoclonic_absences.html. Last accessed 12 Aug 2011.
83. Elia M, Guerrini R, Musumeci SA, Bonanni P, Gambardella A, Aguglia U. Myoclonic absence-like seizures and chromosome abnormality syndromes. Epilepsia. 1998;39:660–3.
84. Ferrie CD, Giannakodimos S, Robinson RO, Panayiotopoulos CP. Symptomatic typical absence seizures. In: Duncan JS, Panayiotopoulos CP, editors. Typical absences and related epileptic syndromes. London: Churchill Communications Europe; 1995. p. 241–52.
85. Tassinari CA, Michelucci R, Rubboli G, Passarelli D, Riguzzi P, Parmeggiani L. Myoclonic absence epilepsy. In: Duncan JS, Panayiotopoulos CP, editors. Typical absences and related epileptic syndromes. London: Churchill Communications Europe; 1995. p. 187–95.
86. Hirsch E, Thomas P, Panayiotopoulos CP. Childhood and juvenile absence epilepsies. In: Jr Engel J, Pedley TA, editors. Epilepsy: a comprehensive textbook. 2nd ed. Phlladelphia: Lippincott William and Wilkins; 2008. p. 2397–411.
87. Wolf P. Juvenile absence epilepsy. In: Roger J, Bureau M, Dravet C, et al., editors. Epileptic syndromes in infancy, childhood and adolescence. London: John Libbey & Co. Ltd; 1992. p. 307–12.
88. Obeid T. Clinical and genetic aspects of juvenile absence epilepsy. J Neurol. 1994;241:487–91.

89. Panayiotopoulos CP, Giannakodimos S, Chroni E. Typical absences in adults. In: Duncan JS, Panayiotopoulos CP, editors. Typical absences and related epileptic syndromes. London: Churchill Communications Europe; 1995. p. 289–99.
90. Osservatorio Regionale per L'Epilessia (OREp), Lombardy. ILAE classification of epilepsies: its applicability and practical value of different diagnostic categories. Epilepsia. 1996;37:1051–9.
91. Doose H, Volzke E, Scheffner D. Verlaufsformen kindlicher epilepsien mit spike wave-absences. Arch Psychiatr Nervenkr. 1965;207:394–415.
92. Oller L. Prospective study of the differences between the syndromes of infantile absence epilepsy and syndromes of juvenile absence epilepsy. Rev Neurol. 1996;24:930–6.
93. Panayiotopoulos CP. Absence status epilepticus. In: Gilman S, editor. Medlink neurology. San Diego SA: Arbor Publishing Corp; 2009.
94. Agathonikou A, Panayiotopoulos CP, Giannakodimos S, Koutroumanidis M. Typical absence status in adults: diagnostic and syndromic considerations. Epilepsia. 1998;39:1265–76.
95. Berkovic SF, Howell RA, Hay DA, Hopper JL. Epilepsies in twins. In: Wolf J, editor. Epileptic seizures and syndromes. London: John Libbey & Co. Ltd; 1994. p. 157–64.
96. Bianchi A. and the Italian LAE Collaborative Group. Study of concordance of symptoms in families with absence epilepsies. In: Duncan JS, Panayiotopoulos CP, editors. Typical absences and related epileptic syndromes. London: Churchill Communications Europe; 1995. p. 328–37.
97. Durner M, Zhou G, Fu D, Abreu P, Shinnar S, Resor SR, et al. Evidence for linkage of adolescent-onset idiopathic generalized epilepsies to chromosome 8 and genetic heterogeneity. Am J Hum Genet. 1999;64:1411–9.
98. Sander T, Hildmann T, Kretz R, Furst R, Sailer U, Bauer G, et al. Allelic association of juvenile absence epilepsy with a GluR5 kainate receptor gene (GRIK1) polymorphism. Am J Med Genet. 1997;74: 416–21.
99. Durner M, Keddache MA, Tomasini L, Shinnar S, Resor SR, Cohen J, et al. Genome scan of idiopathic generalized epilepsy: evidence for major susceptibility gene and modifying genes influencing the seizure type. Ann Neurol. 2001;49:328–35.
100. Meencke HJ, Janz D. The significance of microdysgenesia in primary generalized epilepsy: an answer to the considerations of Lyon and Gastaut. Epilepsia. 1985;26:368–71.
101. Woermann FG, Sisodiya SM, Free SL, Duncan JS. Quantitative MRI in patients with idiopathic generalized epilepsy. Evidence of widespread cerebral structural changes. Brain. 1998;121:1661–7.
102. Panayiotopoulos CP, Chroni E, Daskalopoulos C, Baker A, Rowlinson S, Walsh P. Typical absence seizures in adults: clinical, EEG, video-EEG findings and diagnostic/syndromic considerations. J Neurol Neurosurg Psychiatr. 1992;55:1002–8.
103. Berkovic SF, Knowlton RC, Leroy RF, Schiemann J, Falter U. Placebo-controlled study of levetiracetam in idiopathic generalized epilepsy. Neurology. 2007;69:1751–60.
104. Noachtar S, Andermann E, Meyvisch P, Andermann F, Gough WB, Schiemann-Delgado J. Levetiracetam for the treatment of idiopathic generalized epilepsy with myoclonic seizures. Neurology. 2008;70:607–16.
105. Di Bonaventura C, Fattouch J, Mari F, et al. Clinical experience with levetiracetam in idiopathic generalized epilepsy according to different syndrome subtypes. Epileptic Disord. 2005;7:231–5.
106. Cavitt J, Privitera M. Levetiracetam induces a rapid and sustained reduction of generalized spike-wave and clinical absence. Arch Neurol. 2004;61:1604–7.
107. Striano P, Sofia V, Capovilla G, et al. A pilot trial of levetiracetam in eyelid myoclonia with absences (Jeavons syndrome). Epilepsia. 2008;49:425–30.
108. Verrotti A, Cerminara C, Domizio S, et al. Levetiracetam in absence epilepsy. Dev Med Child Neurol. 2008;50:850–3.
109. Grunewald RA, Panayiotopoulos CP. Juvenile myoclonic epilepsy. A review Arch Neurol. 1993;50:594–8.
110. Camfield CS, Camfield PR. Juvenile myoclonic epilepsy 25 years after seizure onset: a population-based study. Neurology. 2009;73:1041–5.
111. Kobayashi E, Zifkin BG, Andermann F, Andermann E. Juvenile myoclonic epilepsy. In: Engel Jr J, Pedley TA, editors. Epilepsy: a comprehensive textbook. 2nd ed. Philadelphia: Lippincott William and Wilkins; 2008. p. 2455–60.
112. Panayiotopoulos CP, Obeid T, Tahan AR. Juvenile myoclonic epilepsy: a 5-year prospective study. Epilepsia. 1994;35:285–96.
113. Genton P, Gelisse P. Juvenile myoclonic epilepsy. Arch Neurol. 2001;58:1487–90.
114. Janz D, Christian W. [Impulsiv-petit mal.] Z Nervenheilk 1957;176:346–386 (Translated into English by P Genton.). In: Malafosse A, P Genton, E Hirsch, Marescaux C, Broglin D, Bernasconi R, editors. Idiopathic generalised epilepsies. London: John Libbey & Co. Ltd; 1994. p. 229–51.
115. Delgado-Escueta AV, Enrile-Bacsal F. Juvenile myoclonic epilepsy of Janz. Neurology. 1984;34:285–94.
116. Panayiotopoulos CP. Juvenile myoclonic epilepsy: an uderdiagnosed syndrome. In: Wolf P, editor. Epileptic seizures and syndromes. London: John Libbey & Co. Ltd; 1994. p. 221–30.

117. Oguni H, Mukahira K, Oguni M, Uehara T, Su YH, Izumi T, et al. Video-polygraphic analysis of myoclonic seizures in juvenile myoclonic epilepsy. Epilepsia. 1994;35:307–16.
118. Panayiotopoulos CP, Obeid T, Waheed G. Absences in juvenile myoclonic epilepsy: a clinical and video-electroencephalographic study. Ann Neurol. 1989;25:391–7.
119. Canevini MP, Mai R, Di Marco C, Bertin C, Minotti L, Pontrelli V, et al. Juvenile myoclonic epilepsy of Janz: clinical observations in 60 patients. Seizure. 1992;1:291–8.
120. Salas Puig J, Tunon A, Vidal JA, Mateos V, Guisasola LM, Lahoz CH. Janz's juvenile myoclonic epilepsy: a little-known frequent syndrome. A study of 85 patients. Med Clin (Barc). 1994;103:684–9.
121. Pascalicchio TF, Araujo Filho GM, Da Silva Noffs MH, Lin K, Caboclo LOSF, Vidal-Dourado M, et al. Neuropsychological profile of patients with juvenile myoclonic epilepsy: a controlled study of 50 patients. Epilepsy Behav. 2007;10:263–7.
122. Valeta T. Personality, behavioural, cognitive and psychological features of juvenile myoclonic epilepsy. In: Panayiotopoulos CP, editor. Idiopathic generalised epilepsies with myoclonic jerks, vol. 2. Oxford: Medicinae; 2007. p. 66–71.
123. de Araujo Filho GM, Jackowski AP, Lin K. Personality traits related to juvenile myoclonic epilepsy: MRI reveals prefrontal abnormalities through a voxel-based morphometry study. Epilepsy Behav. 2009;15:202–7.
124. Karachristianou S, Katsarou Z, Bostantjopoulou S, Economou A, Garyfallos G, Delinikopoulou E. Personality profile of patients with juvenile myoclonic epilepsy. Epilepsy Behav. 2008;13:654–7.
125. Panayiotopoulos CP, Obeid T. Juvenile myoclonic epilepsy: an autosomal recessive disease. Ann Neurol. 1989;25:440–3.
126. Janz D. Juvenile myoclonic epilepsy. Epilepsy with impulsive petit mal. Cleve Clin J Med. 1989;56(Suppl):S23–33; discussion:S40–2.
127. Serratosa JM, Delgado-Escueta AV, Medina MT, Zhang Q, Iranmanesh R, Sparkes RS. Clinical and genetic analysis of a large pedigree with juvenile myoclonic epilepsy. Ann Neurol. 1996;39:187–95.
128. Tsuboi T, Christian W. On the genetics of the primary generalised epilepsy with sporadic myoclonus of impulsive petit mal type. Humangenetik. 1973;19:155–82.
129. Delgado-Escueta AV, Medina MT, Serratosa JM, Castroviejo IP, Gee MN, Weissbecker K, et al. Mapping and positional cloning of common idiopathic generalized epilepsies: juvenile myoclonus epilepsy and childhood absence epilepsy. Adv Neurol. 1999;79:351–74.
130. Delgado-Escueta AV, Greenberg D, Weissbecker K, Liu A, Treiman L, Sparkes R, et al. Gene mapping in the idiopathic generalized epilepsies: juvenile myoclonic epilepsy, childhood absence epilepsy, epilepsy with grand mal seizures, and early childhood myoclonic epilepsy. Epilepsia. 1990;31 Suppl 3:S19–29.
131. Elmslie FV, Rees M, Williamson MP, Kerr M, Kjeldsen MJ, Pang KA, et al. Genetic mapping of a major susceptibility locus for juvenile myoclonic epilepsy on chromosome 15q. Hum Mol Genet. 1997;6:1329–34.
132. Taske NL, Williamson MP, Makoff A, Bate L, Curtis D, Kerr M, et al. Evaluation of the positional candidate gene CHRNA7 at the juvenile myoclonic epilepsy locus (EJM2) on chromosome 15q13-14. Epilepsy Res. 2002;49:157–72.
133. Suzuki T, Ganesh S, Agarwala KL, Morita R, Sugimoto Y, Inazawa J, et al. A novel gene in the chromosomal region for juvenile myoclonic epilepsy on 6p12 encodes a brain-specific lysosomal membrane protein. Biochem Biophys Res Commun. 2001;288:626–36.
134. Greenberg DA, Durner M, Shinnar S, Resor S, Rosenbaum D, Klotz I, et al. Association of HLA class II alleles in patients with juvenile myoclonic epilepsy compared with patients with other forms of adolescent-onset generalized epilepsy. Neurology. 1996;47:750–5.
135. Obeid T, el Rab MO, Daif AK, Panayiotopoulos CP, Halim K, Bahakim H, et al. Is HLA-DRW13 (W6) associated with juvenile myoclonic epilepsy in Arab patients? Epilepsia. 1994;35:319–21.
136. Le Hellard S, Neidhart E, Thomas P, Feingold J, Malafosse A, Tafti M. Lack of association between juvenile myoclonic epilepsy and HLADR13. Epilepsia. 1999;40:117–9.
137. Koepp MJ. Juvenile myoclonic epilepsy – a generalized epilepsy syndrome? Acta Neurol Scand Suppl. 2005;181:57–62.
138. Woermann FG, Free SL, Koepp MJ, Woermann FG, Free SL, Koepp MJ. Abnormal cerebral structure in juvenile myoclonic epilepsy demonstrated with voxel-based analysis of MRI. Brain. 1999;122:2101–8.
139. Panayiotopoulos CP, Tahan R, Obeid T. Juvenile myoclonic epilepsy: factors of error involved in the diagnosis and treatment. Epilepsia. 1991;32:672–6.
140. Grunewald RA, Chroni E, Panayiotopoulos CP. Delayed diagnosis of juvenile myoclonic epilepsy. J Neurol Neurosurg Psychiatr. 1992;55:497–9.
141. Wirrell EC, Camfield CS, Camfield PR, Gordon KE, Dooley JM. Longterm prognosis of typical childhood absence epilepsy: remission or progression to juvenile myoclonic epilepsy. Neurology. 1996;47:912–8.
142. Anonymous. Diagnosing juvenile myoclonic epilepsy. Lancet. 1992;340:759–60.
143. Baykan B, Altindag EA, Bebek N, Ozturk AY, Aslantas B, et al. Myoclonic seizures subside in the fourth decade in juvenile myoclonic epilepsy. Neurology. 2008;70:2123–9.

144. Penry JK, Dean JC, Riela AR. Juvenile myoclonic epilepsy: long-term response to therapy. Epilepsia. 1989;30 Suppl 4:19–23; discussion: S24–7.
145. Gelisse P, Genton P, Thomas P, Rey M, Samuelian JC, Dravet C. Clinical factors of drug resistance in juvenile myoclonic epilepsy. J Neurol Neurosurg Psychiatr. 2001;70:240–3.
146. Verrotti A, Cerminara C, Coppola G, Franzoni E, Parisi P, et al. Levetiracetam in juvenile myoclonic epilepsy: long-term efficacy in newly diagnosed adolescents. Dev Med Child Neurol. 2008;50:29–32.
147. Sharpe DV, Patel AD, Abou-Khalil B, Fenichel GM. Levetiracetam monotherapy in juvenile myoclonic epilepsy. Seizure. 2008;17:64–8.
148. Abou-Khalil BW. Levetiracetam efficacy in idiopathic generalized epilepsy: long suspected and now confirmed in randomized clinical trials. Epilepsy Curr. 2008;8:16–8.
149. Grunewald R. Levetiracetam in the treatment of idiopathic generalized epilepsies. Epilepsia. 2005;46 Suppl 9:154–60.
150. Biraben A, Allain H, Scarabin JM, Schuck S, Edan G. Exacerbation of juvenile myoclonic epilepsy with lamotrigine. Neurology. 2000;55:1758.
151. Crespel A, Genton P, Berramdane M, Coubes P, Monicard C, Baldy-Moulinier M, et al. Lamotrigine associated with exacerbation or de novo myoclonus in idiopathic generalized epilepsies. Neurology. 2005;65:762–4.
152. Crawford P. Best practice guidelines for the management of women with epilepsy. Epilepsia. 2005;46 Suppl 9:117–24.
153. Petrenaite V, Sabers A, Hansen-Schwartz J. Individual changes in lamotrigine plasma concentrations during pregnancy. Epilepsy Res. 2005;65:185–8.
154. de Haan GJ, Edelbroek P, Segers J, Engelsman M, Lindhout D, Devile-Notschaele M, et al. Gestation-induced changes in lamotrigine pharmacokinetics: a monotherapy study. Neurology. 2004;63:571–3.
155. Pennell PB, Newport DJ, Stowe ZN, Helmers SL, Montgomery JQ, Henry TR. The impact of pregnancy and childbirth on the metabolism of lamotrigine. Neurology. 2004;62:292–5.
156. Holmes LB, Wyszynski DF, Baldwin EJ, Haebecker E, Glassman LH, Smith CR. Increased risk for non-syndromic cleft palate among infants exposed to lamotrigine during pregnancy. Birth Defects Res A Clin Mol Teratol. 2006;76:318.
157. Obeid T, Panayiotopoulos CP. Clonazepam in juvenile myoclonic epilepsy. Epilepsia. 1989;30:603–6.
158. Wolf P. Epilepsy with grand mal on awakening. In: Roger J, Bureau M, Dravet C, editors. Epileptic syndromes in infancy, childhood and adolescence. London: John Libbey & Co. Ltd; 1992. p. 329–41.
159. Panayiotopoulos CP, Koutroumanidis M, Giannakodimos S, Agathonikou A. Idiopathic generalised epilepsy in adults manifested by phantom absences, generalised tonic-clonic seizures, and frequent absence status. J Neurol Neurosurg Psychiatr. 1997;63:622–7.
160. Koutroumanidis M, Aggelakis K, Panayiotopoulos CP. Idiopathic epilepsy with generalized tonic-clonic seizures only versus idiopathic epilepsy with phantom absences and generalized tonic-clonic seizures: one or two syndromes? Epilepsia. 2008;49:2050–62.
161. Roger J, Bureau M, Oller Ferrer-Vidal L, Oller Daurella T, Saltarelli A, Genton P. Clinical and electroencephalographic characteristics of idiopathic generalised epilepsies. In: Malafosse A, Genton P, Hirsch E, Marescaux C, Broglin D, Bernasconi R, editors. Idiopathic generalised epilepsies. London: John Libbey & Co. Ltd; 1994. p. 7–18.
162. Oller-Daurella LF-V, Oller L. 5000 Epilepticos. Clinica y Evolucion. Barcelona, Spain: Ciba-Geigy; 1994.
163. Janz D. Epilepsy with grand mal on awakening and sleep-waking cycle. Clin Neurophysiol. 2000;111 Suppl 2:S103–10.
164. Janz D. Pitfalls in the diagnosis of grand mal on awakening. In: Wolf P, editor. Epileptic seizures and syndromes. London: John Libbey & Co. Ltd; 1994. p. 213–20.
165. Janz D. Die epilepsien: spezielle pathologie and therapie. Stuttgart: Georg Thieme; 1969.
166. Greenberg DA, Durner M, Resor S, Rosenbaum D, Shinnar S. The genetics of idiopathic generalized epilepsies of adolescent onset: differences between juvenile myoclonic epilepsy and epilepsy with random grand mal and with awakening grand mal. Neurology. 1995;45:942–6.
167. Berg A, Blackstone NW. Reply to "Of cabbages and kings: some considerations on classifications, diagnostic schemes, semiology, and concepts". Epilepsia. 2003;44:8–12.
167a. Leen WG, Klepper J, Verbeek MM, et al. Glucose transporter-1 deficiency syndrome: the expanding clinical and genetic spectrum of a treatable disorder. Brain 2010;133:655–70.
167b. Striano P, Weber YG, Toliat MR et al. GLUT1 mutations are a rare cause of familial idiopathic generalized epilepsy. Neurology 2012;78:557–62.
168. Rubboli G, Gardella E, Capovilla G. Idiopathic generalized epilepsy (IGE) syndromes in development: IGE with absences of early childhood, IGE with phantom absences, and perioral myoclonia with absences. Epilepsia. 2009;50 Suppl 5:24–8.
169. Genton P, Ferlazzo E, Thomas P. Absence status epilepsy: delineation of a distinct idiopathic generalized epilepsy syndrome. Epilepsia. 2008;49:642–9.
170. Baier WK, Doose H. Petit mal-absences of childhood onset: familial prevalences of migraine and seizures. Neuropediatrics. 1985;16:80–3.

171. Doose H. Absence epilepsy of early childhood – genetic aspects. Eur J Pediatr. 1994;153:372–7.

172. Doose H. Absence epilepsy of early childhood. In: Wolf P, editor. Epileptic seizures and syndromes. London: John Libbey & Co. Ltd; 1994. p. 133–5.

173. Fernandez-Torre JL, Herranz JL, Martinez-Martinez M, Maestro I, Arteaga R, Barrasa J. Early-onset absence epilepsy: clinical and electroencephalographic features in three children. Brain Dev. 2006;28:311–4.

174. Panayiotopoulos CP, Ferrie CD, Giannakodimos S, Robinson RO. Perioral myoclonia with absences: a new syndrome. In: Wolf P, editor. Epileptic seizures and syndromes. London: John Libbey & Co. Ltd; 1994. p. 143–53.

175. Panayiotopoulos CP. Typical absence seizures. In: Gilman S, editor. Medlink neurology. San Diego, CA: Arbor Publishing Corp; 2007.

176. Clemens B. Perioral myoclonia with absences? A case report with EEG and voltage mapping analysis. Brain Dev. 1997;19:353–8.

177. Bilgic B, Baykan B, Gurses C, Gokyigit A. Perioral myoclonia with absence seizures: a rare epileptic syndrome. Epileptic Disord. 2001;3:23–7.

178. Capovilla G, Rubboli G, Beccaria F, Lorenzetti ME, Montagnini A, Resi C, et al. A clinical spectrum of the myoclonic manifestations associated with typical absences in childhood absence epilepsy. A video-polygraphic study. Epileptic Disord. 2001;3:57–62.

179. Baykan B, Noachtar S. Perioral myoclonia with absences: an overlooked and misdiagnosed generalized seizure type. Epilepsy Behav. 2005;6:460–2.

180. Panayiotopoulos CP. Typical absences are syndrome related. In: Duncan JS, Panayiotopoulos CP, editors. Typical absences and related epileptic syndromes. London: Churchill Communications Europe; 1995. p. 304–10.

181. Genton P. Epilepsy with 3Hz spike-and-waves without clinically evident absences. In: Duncan JS, Panayiotopoulos CP, editors. Typical absences and related epileptic syndromes. London: Churchill Communications Europe; 1995. p. 231–8.

182. Panayiotopoulos CP. Epilepsy with generalised tonic-clonic seizures on awakening. In: Wallace S, editor. Epilepsy in children. London: Chapman & Hall; 1996. p. 349–53.

183. Marini C, King MA, Archer JS, Newton MR, Berkovic SF. Idiopathic generalised epilepsy of adult onset: clinical syndromes and genetics. J Neurol Neurosurg Psychiatr. 2003;74:192–6.

184. Nicolson A, Chadwick DW, Smith DF. A comparison of adult onset and "classical" idiopathic generalised epilepsy. J Neurol Neurosurg Psychiatr. 2004;75:72–4.

185. Striano P, Zara F, Striano S. Autosomal dominant cortical tremor, myoclonus and epilepsy: many syndromes, one phenotype. Acta Neurol Scand. 2005;111:211–7.

186. Guerrini R, Parmeggiani L, Marini C, Brovedani P, Bonanni P. Autosomal dominant cortical myoclonus and epilepsy (ADCME) with linkage to chromosome 2p11.1-q12.2. Adv Neurol. 2005;95:273–9.

187. Suppa A, Berardelli A, Brancati F, et al. Clinical, neuropsychological, neurophysiologic, and genetic features of a new Italian pedigree with familial cortical myoclonic tremor with epilepsy. Epilepsia. 2009;50:1284–8.

188. Magnin E, Vidailhet M, Depienne C, et al. Familial cortical myoclonic tremor with epilepsy (FCMTE): Clinical characteristics and exclusion of linkages to 8q and 2p in a large French family. Rev Neurol (Paris). 2009;165:812–20.

189. Zara F, Gennaro E, Stabile M, Carbone I, Malacarne M, Majello L, et al. Mapping of a locus for a familial autosomal recessive idiopathic myoclonic epilepsy of infancy to chromosome 16p13. Am J Hum Genet. 2000;66:1552–7.

190. de Falco FA, Majello L, Santangelo R, Stabile M, Bricarelli FD, Zara F. Familial infantile myoclonic epilepsy: clinical features in a large kindred with autosomal recessive inheritance. Epilepsia. 2001;42:1541–8.

191. Uyama E, Fu YH, Ptacek LJ. Familial adult myoclonic epilepsy (FAME). Adv Neurol. 2005;95:281–8.

192. Shibasaki H, Hallett M. Electrophysiological studies of myoclonus. Muscle Nerve. 2005;31:157–74.

193. Mikami M, Yasuda T, Terao A, Nakamura M, Ueno S, Tanabe H, et al. Localization of a gene for benign adult familial myoclonic epilepsy to chromosome 8q23.3-q24.1. Am J Hum Genet. 1999;65:745–51.

194. Plaster NM, Uyama E, Uchino M, Ikeda T, Flanigan KM, Kondo I, et al. Genetic localization of the familial adult myoclonic epilepsy (FAME) gene to chromosome 8q24. Neurology. 1999;53:1180–3.

195. Labauge P, Amer LO, Simonetta-Moreau M, Attane F, Tannier C, Clanet M, et al. Absence of linkage to 8q24 in a European family with familial adult myoclonic epilepsy (FAME). Neurology. 2002;58:941–4.

196. Striano P, Manganelli F, Boccella P, Perretti A, Striano S. Levetiracetam in patients with cortical myoclonus: a clinical and electrophysiological study. Mov Disord. 2005;20:1610–4.

196a. Panayiotopoulos CP. A Clinical Guide to Epileptic Syndromes and Their Treatment. Revised 2nd edition. London: Springer, 2010

197. French JA, Kanner AM, Bautista J, Abou Khalil B, Browne T, Harden CL, et al. Efficacy and tolerability of the new antiepileptic drugs I: treatment of new onset epilepsy: report of the Therapeutics and Technology Assessment Subcommittee and Quality Standards Subcommittee of the American Academy of Neurology and the American Epilepsy Society. Neurology. 2004;62:1252–60.

198. Zaccara G, Gangemi PF, Cincotta M. Central nervous system adverse effects of new antiepileptic drugs. A meta-analysis of placebo-controlled studies. Seizure. 2008;17:405–21.
199. Patsalos PN. Anti-epileptic drug interactions: a clinical guide. Cranleigh, UK: Clarius Press Ltd; 2005.
200. Guerrini R, Dravet C, Genton P, Belmonte A, Kaminska A, Dulac O. Lamotrigine and seizure aggravation in severe myoclonic epilepsy. Epilepsia. 1998;39:508–12.
201. Guerrini R, Belmonte A, Parmeggiani L, Perucca E. Myoclonic status epilepticus following high-dosage lamotrigine therapy. Brain Dev. 1999;21:420–4.
202. Faught E. Clinical trials for treatment of primary generalized epilepsies. Epilepsia. 2003;44 Suppl 7:44–50.
203. Sundqvist A, Nilsson BY, Tomson T. Valproate monotherapy in juvenile myoclonic epilepsy: dose-related effects on electroencephalographic and other neurophysiologic tests. Ther Drug Monit. 1999;21:91–6.
204. Glauser T, Ben-Menachem E, Bourgeois B, Cnaan A, Chadwick D, Guerreiro C, et al. ILAE treatment guidelines: evidence-based analysis of antiepileptic drug efficacy and effectiveness as initial monotherapy for epileptic seizures and syndromes. Epilepsia. 2006;47:1094–120.
205. Biton V, Montouris GD, Ritter F, Riviello JJ, Reife R, Lim P, et al. A randomized, placebo-controlled study of topiramate in primary generalized tonic-clonic seizures. Topiramate YTC Study Group. Neurology. 1999;52:1330–7.
206. Marson AG, Al-Kharusi AM, Alwaidh M, Appleton R, Baker GA, Chadwick DW, et al. The SANAD study of effectiveness of valproate, lamotrigine, or topiramate for generalised and unclassifiable epilepsy: an unblinded randomised controlled trial. Lancet. 2007;369:1016–26.
207. Muller M, Marson AG, Williamson PR. Oxcarbazepine versus phenytoin monotherapy for epilepsy. Cochrane Database Syst Rev. 2006;2:CD003615.
208. French JA. First-choice drug for newly diagnosed epilepsy. Lancet. 2007;369:970–1.
209. Cunnington M, Tennis P. Lamotrigine and the risk of malformations in pregnancy. Neurology. 2005;64:955–60.
210. Morrow J, Russell A, Guthrie E, Parsons L, Robertson I, Waddell R, et al. Malformation risks of antiepileptic drugs in pregnancy: a prospective study from the UK Epilepsy and Pregnancy Register. J Neurol Neurosurg Psychiatr. 2006;77:193–8.
211. Resor Jr SR, Resor LD. Chronic acetazolamide monotherapy in the treatment of juvenile myoclonic epilepsy. Neurology. 1990;40:1677–81.
212. Rosenfeld WE, Benbadis S, Edrich P, Tassinari CA, Hirsch E. Levetiracetam as add-on therapy for idiopathic generalized epilepsy syndromes with onset during adolescence: analysis of two randomized, double-blind, placebo-controlled studies. Epilepsy Res. 2009;85:72–80.
213. Lyseng-Williamson KA. Levetiracetam: a review of its use in epilepsy. Drugs 2011;71:489–514.
214. Hunt S, Craig J, Russell A, Guthrie E, Parsons L, Robertson I, et al. Levetiracetam in pregnancy: preliminary experience from the UK Epilepsy and Pregnancy Register. Neurology. 2006;67:1876–9.
215. Biton V, Sackellares JC, Vuong A, Hammer AE, Barrett PS, Messenheimer JA. Double-blind, placebo-controlled study of lamotrigine in primary generalized tonic-clonic seizures. Neurology. 2005;65:1737–43.
216. Tran TA, Leppik IE, Blesi K, Sathanandan ST, Remmel R. Lamotrigine clearance during pregnancy. Neurology. 2002;59:251–5.
217. Sabers A, Ohman I, Christensen J, Tomson T. Oral contraceptives reduce lamotrigine plasma levels. Neurology. 2003;61:570–1.
218. Privitera MD. Topiramate. In: Wyllie E, Gupta A, Lachhwani D, editors. The treatment of epilepsy: principles and practice. 4th ed. Philadelphia: Lippincott Williams & Wilkins; 2006. p. 877–89.
219. Cross JH. Topiramate monotherapy for childhood absence seizures: an open label pilot study. Seizure. 2002;11:406–10.
220. Kjellstrom S, Bruun A, Isaksson B, Eriksson T, Andreasson S, Ponjavic V. Retinal function and histopathology in rabbits treated with topiramate. Doc Ophthalmol. 2006;113:179–86.
221. Panayiotopoulos CP. Juvenile myoclonic epilepsy. In: Panayiotopoulos CP, editor. The epilepsies: seizures, syndromes and management. Updated reprint. Oxford: Bladon Medical Publishing; 2005. p. 1–24.
222. Baulac M. Introduction to zonisamide. Epilepsy Res. 2006;68 Suppl 2:S3–9.
223. French JA, Kanner AM, Bautista J, Abou-Khalil B, Browne T, Harden CL, et al. Efficacy and tolerability of the new antiepileptic drugs, II: treatment of refractory epilepsy: report of the TTA and QSS Subcommittees of the American Academy of Neurology and the American Epilepsy Society. Epilepsia. 2004;45:410–23.
224. Siren A, Eriksson K, Jalava H, Kilpinen-Loisa P, Koivikko M. Idiopathic generalised epilepsies with 3 Hz and faster spike wave discharges: a population-based study with evaluation and long-term follow-up in 71 patients. Epileptic Disord. 2002;4:209–16.
225. Panayiotopoulos C.P. Absence status epilepticus. http://www.ilae-epilepsy.org/Visitors/Centre/ctf/absence_status_epilepticus.html. Last accessed 12 Aug 2011.

Index

A

Absence(s) (absence seizures; petit mal)
  AED treatment, 61–63
  childhood (CAE), 13–20
    classification, 13–16
    differential diagnosis, 18–19, 23
    in Doose syndrome, 6
    idiopathic generalised epilepsy with
      in early childhood, 47
      phantom absences, 53–57
    myoclonic, 21–24
    perioral myoclonia with, 49–51
    typical (TAS), 14, 16
      in IGE with phantom absences, 54
      in juvenile absence epilepsy, 26
      in juvenile myoclonic epilepsy,
        31–35
      with perioral myoclonia, 49
Absence status epilepticus, 45
  in IGE with phantom absences, 54, 55
  in juvenile absence epilepsy, 27, 29
  in perioral myoclonia with absences,
    50, 51
Acetazolamide and idiopathic
    generalised epilepsies, 67
Adolescence, juvenile absence epilepsy
    vs. myoclonic epilepsy in, 28
Adrenocorticotrophic hormone (ACTH)
    and Lennox–Gastaut syndrome,
    24
Antiepileptic drugs (AEDs;
    anticonvulsants)
  evidence-based recommendations in
    idiopathic generalised epilepsy,
    65–67
  in idiopathic generalised epilepsy/IGE
    (in general), 61–70
    contraindicated, 40, 61–63, 69, 70
    newer AEDs, 68 69
    newly diagnosed IGEs, 65, 66

older AEDs, 67–68
withdrawal, 20, 40, 69, 70
prophylaxis in generalised
    tonic–clonic seizures, 65
resistance (intractable/refractory/
    difficult-to-treat epilepsy) in
    idiopathic generalised epilepsy,
    69–70
withdrawal/discontinuance/stopping
    with absence epilepsy in childhood, 20
    with idiopathic generalised
      epilepsies, 20, 40, 69, 70
Atonic seizures in Doose syndrome, 6
Atypical benign partial epilepsy (APEC),
    10
Automatisms in childhood absence
    epilepsy, 19
Autosomal dominant conditions in
    juvenile myoclonic epilepsy, 35

B

Benign epileptic seizures (children), 10

C

Carbamazepine
  idiopathic generalised epilepsies
    contraindications, 32, 64, 67
    generalised tonic–clonic seizures, 64,
      67
  juvenile myoclonic epilepsy, erroneous
    use and contraindication, 32
Chromosome 6 open reading frame 33
    (*C6orf33*), 35
Circadian distribution
  juvenile absence epilepsy, 28
  juvenile myoclonic epilepsy, 28, 34–35
Clonazepam
  generalised tonic–clonic seizures, 63,
    65, 67